Comprehensive Clinical Care for Adolescents with Avoidant/Restrictive Food Intake Disorder (ARFID)

Anne B. Sinha • Allyson F. Sy
Jennifer L. Derenne • Jennifer L. Carlson

Comprehensive Clinical Care for Adolescents with Avoidant/Restrictive Food Intake Disorder (ARFID)

A Multidisciplinary Approach

Springer

Anne B. Sinha
Occupational Therapy Rehabilitation Services
Stanford Medicine Children's Health, Lucile Packard Children's Hospital
Palo Alto, CA, USA

Jennifer L. Derenne
Child and Adolescent Psychiatry
Stanford University
Palo Alto, CA, USA

Allyson F. Sy
Clinical Nutrition Services
The Healthy Teen Project, San Francisco
San Francisco, CA, USA

Jennifer L. Carlson
Adolescent Medicine
Stanford University
Palo Alto, CA, USA

ISBN 978-3-031-92231-2 ISBN 978-3-031-92232-9 (eBook)
https://doi.org/10.1007/978-3-031-92232-9

This Springer imprint is published by the registered company Springer Nature Switzerland AG
The registered company address is: Gewerbestrasse 11, 6330 Cham, Switzerland

Foreword

Why write a book about Avoidant Restrictive Food Intake Disorder (ARFID)? Many families who have come into our care report working with a multidisciplinary team, various medical and/or naturopathic practitioners, and other institutions for treatment, yet many have not yet found a sustainable solution for their child's unique eating problems.

We are excited to share what we have done as a treatment team in hopes of inspiring other professionals to do the same or, at the very least, be inspired to explore on your own how to best treat individuals with ARFID. Throughout the years of our clinical work, we discovered that every person with ARFID is unique and that a single approach would not be sufficiently effective for the variety of patients we meet. We adapted our treatment protocols and iterated on our management tools to develop a much more individualized and holistic approach with the goals of improving patient care. While some of the strategies may be widely used, evidence-based techniques, other tools may seem more unique as they have been developed within our program. We have attempted to clearly identify when a tool or strategy is one associated with our program or our authors. We recognize the need to study various interventions in the future.

It is important to acknowledge our privileges and the benefits of having a well-funded, specialized, eating disorder focused inpatient unit. We are fortunate to have a team composed of experienced clinicians and a well-staffed organization. We have spoken with other clinicians from around the world and know that many organizations, hospitals, and practices are not as well equipped. With that awareness in mind, we hope that with this book, you can learn how to connect to other health professionals and learn to best manage your current resources.

Within the chapters, you will find specific information presented by each of our disciplines. You may notice that many of the same themes or suggestions are mentioned in each of the individual chapters, highlighting just how useful it is to have a multidisciplinary team with whom you can collaborate. The second part of the book is a series of cases in which we apply the skills and recommendations that we previously introduced. While each case has been altered to protect patient privacy, all cases are based on an amalgam of our real-life experience. Finally, we have included many of our tools in the Appendix for your management of patients with ARFID.

After years of direct experience with thousands of patients, this professional team has adapted and developed recommendations that can enable recovery from ARFID. This book is written with the hope that more practitioners will be able to treat patients as effectively and promptly as possible utilizing new techniques and/or approaches to care. We hope that more children, adolescents, and young adults (and their families!) will achieve their best possible health, one that reopens the door to participation in typical daily activities, as well as future life opportunities.

Palo Alto, CA, USA — Anne B. Sinha
San Francisco, CA, USA — Allyson F. Sy
Palo Alto, CA, USA — Jennifer L. Derenne
Palo Alto, CA, USA — Jennifer L. Carlson

Acknowledgments

First, we would like to express our sincere gratitude to our patients and their families for entrusting us with their care which ultimately paved the way to help formulate our current recommendations. Watching patients grow and thrive over the years, across different levels of care, has been an extraordinary privilege.

Our heartfelt thanks also go to the incredible Stanford Children team members whose dedication has been essential to this work. Your consultations, support, and adaptability have been vital in the implementation and success of these interventions. To our inpatient and clinical partners, including nurses, milieu teams, and adolescent medicine physicians, whose patience, adaptability, and steadfast commitment have been foundational.

Special acknowledgment goes to Kelley Davis, RD, for invaluable dietary mentorship, and to Patrick Rodriguez, DTR, for the tireless support in bringing meal plans to life, ensuring no detail was overlooked. Special appreciation to occupational therapist Marianna Thorn, whose foundational work in feeding informed the OT ARFID approach, and to nurse practitioner Diana Sherman, whose collaboration helped make Occupational Therapy Feeding Plans viable and effective.

The unwavering support of our families, children, and friends has been invaluable, allowing us to embark on this demanding yet rewarding journey. So much becomes possible when others believe in you.

Finally, this book is a tribute to each of you who have shaped and supported our mission to advance ARFID care. It is our hope that this work will honor your contributions and further empower others in the field.

Contents

About the Authors

Anne B. Sinha is a seasoned pediatric occupational therapist with 25 years of experience. For the past 19 years she has specialized in eating disorder treatment at Stanford Children's Hospital. She holds an SWC (advanced practice certification in Swallowing Assessment, Evaluation, or Intervention) from the California Board of Occupational Therapy. Anne has made a significant impact through her work in both inpatient and outpatient settings. She is known for her innovative approaches that advance ARFID treatment. She is currently developing an application for ARFID patients and has developed multiple educational videos referenced and available within this publication. Beyond her professional life, Anne enjoys spending time in nature with her husband and three boys, reading, and practicing breathing techniques.

Allyson F. Sy MS, RD, has worked primarily in eating disorders for the past 10 years and currently works as the director of nutrition at an adolescent eating disorder clinic and sees clients in her private practice. She previously worked for Stanford Children's Health, most notably as the lead dietitian for the specialized eating disorders inpatient unit, the Comprehensive Care Program, from 2016 to 2019.

Ally remains committed in advancing the field and has published research articles on illness severity in atypical anorexia nervosa and higher-calorie refeeding in anorexia nervosa. She regularly speaks at local and international conferences and events, especially on ARFID nutrition care and management.

She loves spending time with her husband, family, and friends and especially enjoys hiking, yoga, traveling, and discovering the best food the world has to offer.

Jennifer L. Derenne is a physician who is board-certified in general adult psychiatry and child and adolescent psychiatry. She has worked with patients with eating disorders across the life span in inpatient, outpatient, and psychiatric higher level of care settings for the past 20 years. She enjoys traveling, cooking, and playing with her dog Scout.

Jennifer L. Carlson is a physician who is board-certified in pediatrics, adolescent medicine, and clinical informatics. For the past 20 years, she has collaborated in the care for adolescents and young adults with eating disorders in the inpatient and ambulatory settings. Outside of work, she enjoys hiking and exploring with her husband and two teenaged boys.

Abbreviations

ADHD	Attention deficit hyperactivity disorder
ADLs	Activities of daily living
ALT	Alanine transaminase
AM	"Ante meridiem," before noon
AN	Anorexia nervosa
ARFID	Avoidant restrictive food intake disorder
ASD	Autism spectrum disorder
ASQ	Ask Suicide-screening Questions
AST	Aspartate transferase
BL	Bristol stool level
BMI	Body mass index
Bmod	Behavior modification
CBC	Complete blood count
CBT	Cognitive behavioral therapy
CDC	Centers for Disease Control and Prevention
COVID	Coronavirus disease
CV	Cardiovascular
DBT	Dialectical behavior therapy
DSM	Diagnostic and Statistical Manual for Mental Disorders
DXA	Dual energy x-ray absorptiometry
EDE	Eating disorders evaluation
EKG	Electrocardiogram
EOE	Eosinophilic esophagitis
ESR	Erythrocyte sedimentation rate
FBI-ARFID	Feelings and Body Investigators—ARFID Division
FBT	Family-based treatment
FDA	Food and Drug Administration
FNS	Food neophobia scale
FODMAP	Fermentable oligosaccharides, disaccharides, monosaccharides, and polyols
FSH	Follicle-stimulating hormone

G	Gastric
GAD	Generalized anxiety disorder
GER	Gastroesophageal reflux
GERD	Gastroesophageal reflux disease
GI	Gastrointestinal
IEP	Individual education plan
IOP	Intensive outpatient program
HEENT	Head, eyes, ears, nose, throat
Kcals	Calories
LBP	Ladder block plan
LH	Luteinizing hormone
mBMI	Median body mass index
MG	Milligrams
NG	Nasogastric
NGT	Nasogastric tube
NIAS	Nine Item ARFID Screen
NICU	Neonatal intensive care unit
OCD	Obsessive compulsive disorder
OT	Occupational therapist
PARDI	Pica, ARFID, and rumination disorder interview
PANS	Pediatric acute-onset neuropsychiatric disorders
PCP	Primary care physician
PHP	Partial hospitalization program
PHQ 9	Patient health questionnaire
PICU	Pediatric intensive care unit
PM	"Post meridiem," after noon
PO	"Per os," by mouth
PT	Physical therapy
pt.	Patient
PTSD	Post-traumatic stress disorder
QTc	Corrected QT interval
RD	Registered dietitian
RDN	Registered dietitian nutritionist
RTC	residential treatment center
SLP	Speech language pathologist
ST	Speech therapist
SNRI	Selective norepinephrine reuptake inhibitor
SPACE	Supportive Parenting for Anxious Childhood Emotions
SSRI	Selective serotonin reuptake inhibitor
TIPP	Temperature, intense exercise, paced breathing, progressive muscle relaxation
TSH	Thyroid-stimulating hormone

List of Figures

List of Tables

Part I
Content Based Chapters

Chapter 1
Introduction to ARFID & ARFID Subtypes

Avoidant Restrictive Food Intake disorder (hereafter referred to as ARFID) was first officially described in the 2013 iteration of the Diagnostic and Statistical Manual for Mental Disorders (DSM-5), but the symptom presentation is not new [1]. Prior to the ARFID diagnosis, many patients may have been diagnosed with eating disorder not otherwise specified, specific phobia, or simply labeled a "picky eater". The DSM-5 describes ARFID as below:

> An eating or feeding disturbance (e.g., apparent lack of interest in eating or food; avoidance based on the sensory characteristics of food; concern about aversive consequences of eating) associated with one (or more) of the following:

1. Significant weight loss (or failure to achieve expected weight gain or faltering growth in children).
2. Significant nutritional deficiency.
3. Dependence on enteral feeding or oral nutritional supplements.
4. Marked interference with psychosocial functioning.

The exact prevalence of ARFID is unknown but thought to have equal distribution in males and females. It typically arises in early childhood, but when left untreated, can persist into adulthood. ARFID can arise in individuals from all racial and ethnic backgrounds and socioeconomic status, and there are commonly other immediate and extended family members who also experience eating challenges. Family dynamics do not cause ARFID, but high criticism, expressed emotion, and challenges setting firm and consistent boundaries may make recovery challenging. ARFID may present alongside other co-occurring mental health conditions and is often seen in patients with autism spectrum disorders, anxiety disorders, attention deficit hyperactivity disorder (ADHD), and obsessive-compulsive disorder (OCD). Acute food refusal can be a hallmark of pediatric autoimmune neuropsychiatric disorders (PANS) as well.

A. B. Sinha et al., *Comprehensive Clinical Care for Adolescents with Avoidant/Restrictive Food Intake Disorder (ARFID)*,
https://doi.org/10.1007/978-3-031-92232-9_1

In more recent years, ARFID has been discussed not as a single entity, but as a disorder with several distinct subtypes which have unique presentations and findings. While the subtypes have not been officially designated within the DSM-5, there are three common subtypes recognized clinically and in the literature [2–4]. While the subtypes are distinct from each other, an individual person can present with characteristics of more than one subtype at the same time. For the purposes of this book, we will use the following categories to note each of the subtypes: Sensory, Low Interest, and Fear of Aversive Consequences.

Patients with ARFID may feel misunderstood by their medical team and family members, as they may be misdiagnosed or have treatment that is not customized to their specific needs. Parents also can be baffled by their children with ARFID, especially those with sensory issues or low interest. At times, the parents themselves may be "foodies" or fantastic chefs and may identify more with a "live to eat" than the "eat to live" philosophy. Due to this difference between their own experience and that of their child, they may consistently be attempting approaches that do not work. Often these youth require more scaffolding and specialized plans developed in concert with a team. Parents themselves may need to make changes in their own behavior and expectations in order to support their child's progress. Time spent with these parents is equally as important as time spent with their child.

ARFID Subtype: Sensory

Example *12-year old Elijah only liked about five foods. However, his parents said he could only eat so much of those foods "because they weren't healthy." Every day they put vegetables on his plate and every day he refused to eat them. When they would go out to eat at one of two restaurants where he was willing to eat, the only thing he would eat was French fries. As he entered his adolescent years, his weight and height failed to track along his previous growth curve.*

In the sensory subtype of ARFID, an individual has limited their nutritional intake due to some sensory aspect(s) of food. The sensory focus can be variable—texture, color, taste, shape, smell—and can often be very specific. For example, a patient may report cutting out a formerly preferred food due to a recipe change (e.g., when a fast food chain changed their chicken nugget recipe to make it lower in fat). Many parents will say that they have spent their child's whole life handling well-meaning suggestions from clinical providers, friends, and family members. Suggestions like "just feed your child a little of everything," or "don't worry, they won't starve if they don't want to eat what you plate" may work for most children but are not effective for individuals with ARFID. Often these parents feel as though they've tried everything to expand their child's diet but haven't been successful.

Patients with the sensory subtype of ARFID may demonstrate rigidity elsewhere in life, in addition to eating. There appears to be a correlation between the sensory-subtype and an autism spectrum diagnosis or obsessive-compulsive disorder [5, 6]. Selective eating may persist throughout adulthood and can cause nutrient deficiencies, depending on the type of selectivity, if not addressed.

Common Characteristics of Sensory Subtype

- Very picky and has specific food preferences
- May focus on food's appearance, color, texture, flavor, smell
- May be impacted by the source of food (restaurant vs home) or may be sensitive to brand or packaging
- May "cycle" through favorite foods
- May experience food "jags" in which favorite foods are eaten repeatedly until the individual "burns out" on that item and will no longer consume it.
- Might be labeled as "super-tasters"
- Sensitive to any (even minor) changes to the food
- Might need to trial a new food more frequently before acceptance of that food
- May prefer eating the same meals every day
- At times may be able to eat a large amount of preferred foods

ARFID Subtype: Low Interest

Example 15*-year-old Lily has never been very interested in food, she "just doesn't think about it." She frequently goes to school without breakfast (as she would rather sleep in), might nibble on some chips at lunch, and doesn't eat until her family puts dinner in front of her in the evening. She might have a night-time snack if her parents give it to her while she is studying. Her parents hoped her eating would improve as she got older, but it seems to be getting tougher.*

ARFID patients, including those with the low interest subtype, may have previously been diagnosed as failure to thrive or failure to gain weight or grow [7]. Often they have demonstrated minimal or decelerated growth, staying on the lower end of the growth charts for weight, stature, and BMI. Patients may report that they rarely feel hungry, do not have a long list of favorite foods, and would prefer to do other activities rather than eat. For those with a lifelong presentation of disinterested eating, most are not flagged for malnutrition until they begin to struggle with the increased nutritional demands of puberty and, thus, are unable to meet their energy needs. This can result in a decrease in weight percentiles, as well as height percentiles, during the adolescent ages.

When asked, most individuals with low-interest ARFID will report that they are someone who "eats to live" rather than a person who "lives to eat." They will find excuses to not eat, take a few bites and report feeling done with the meal, or will go hours without eating anything. They may also struggle to prioritize eating over other activities. This person may not be easily motivated or influenced to eat even when the environment is conducive to food consumption, such as enjoying cake with their peers at a birthday party.

For individuals with a more acute presentation of the low-interest subtype, depression diagnoses can be an underlying etiology, particularly in individuals who might be anhedonic and socially isolated. In addition, individuals with ADHD might have lower interest due to underlying attention issues or as a possible side effect of medication.

Helping individuals with this ARFID subtype realize that eating and appropriate nutrition are necessary to achieve their broader goals and interests is an important step in their treatment.

Common Characteristics of Low Interest Subtype

- **Typically a chronic, lifelong problem, though can have acute presentations**
- May not have favorite foods (but may have strong dislikes)
- May have difficulty explaining why they don't want to eat; may be related to different hormone levels of ghrelin and leptin [8]
- May not be motivated to eat even when others are eating around them
- Rarely will say "I'm hungry"; may get full easily
- May get bored during a meal
- Meals may take a long time to be completed

ARFID Subtype: Fear of Aversive Consequences

Example *10-year-old Riley was a normal eater until his entire family became sick with the flu. While the rest of the family got better and returned to normal eating, Riley continued to say he worried about vomiting and, subsequently, avoided all food other than yogurt tubes.*

ARFID patients with the fear of aversive consequences subtype often have a history of normal eating but experience an event that suddenly makes them extremely fearful. Examples of events that may lead to a fear of aversive consequences include: experiencing vomiting or choking or seeing someone else vomit or choke on a food item, becoming ill with vomiting or abdominal symptoms, or having a food-related allergic reaction. In addition, elimination diets, sometimes at the recommendation of a healthcare provider, can trigger a fear of consuming multiple foods.

Many parents of children with ARFID-fear of aversive consequences subtype will seek guidance from medical professionals due to the abrupt onset of symptoms. Sometimes parents will be advised to practice watchful waiting to see if the child is able to resume previous eating patterns. In cases where the inciting experience is mildly traumatic and the child has been able to intuitively confront and overcome the fear relatively quickly, this advice may work. However, if the event is perceived as more significant, then the subsequent eating patterns may be more challenging to address and may require additional interventions. Anecdotally, intensive work during an inpatient hospitalization can often help shift these patients back to their baseline eating practices. If the patient is not medically unstable such that an inpatient admission would be warranted, then intensive outpatient work can also help individuals break out of the disordered eating patterns.

Common Characteristics of Fear of Aversive Consequences

- Generally, there has been a traumatic event such as vomiting, choking, or anaphylaxis that precedes the eating challenges
- Prior to the eating changes, the patient was likely able to eat normally and grow/develop appropriately
- May have more abrupt weight loss and resultant vital sign instability
- May have traits of high anxiety or rigidity at baseline
- Many are very sensitive to body sensations such as stomachaches or throat fullness

Our team has found that each ARFID subtype may require different treatment approaches; considering the pattern of response for each subtype can help guide initial treatment. In the instances when a patient may present with features of more than one subtype, characteristics from both areas are considered and the treatment plan is configured to triage issues that are of the highest concern.

References

1. American Psychiatric Association. Diagnostic and statistical manual of mental disorders. 5th ed; 2013. https://doi.org/10.1176/appi.books.9780890425596.
2. Zickgraf HF, Lane-Loney S, Essayli JH, Ornstein RM. Further support for diagnostically meaningful ARFID symptom presentations in an adolescent medicine partial hospitalization program. Int J Eat Disord. 2019;52(4):402–9.
3. Sanchez-Cerezo J, Neale J, Julius N, Croudace T, Lynn RM, Hudson LD, Nicholls D. Subtypes of avoidant/restrictive food intake disorder in children and adolescents: a latent class analysis. EClinicalMedicine. 2024;68:102440.
4. Katzman DK, Guimond T, Spettigue W, Agostino H, Couturier J, Norris ML. Classification of children and adolescents with avoidant/restrictive food intake disorder. Pediatrics. 2022;150(3):e2022057494. https://doi.org/10.1542/peds.2022-057494. PMID: 35945342.
5. Farag F, Sims A, Strudwick K, Carrasco J, Waters A, Ford V, Hopkins J, Whitlingum G, Absoud M, Kelly VB. Avoidant/restrictive food intake disorder and autism spectrum disorder: clinical implications for assessment and management. Dev Med Child Neurol. 2022;64(2):176–82.
6. Dovey TM, Kumari V, Blissett J, Mealtime Hostage Parent Science Gang. Eating behaviour, behavioural problems and sensory profiles of children with avoidant/restrictive food intake dis-

order (ARFID), autistic spectrum disorders or picky eating: same or different? Eur Psychiatry. 2019;61:56–62.

7. Dinkler L, Wronski ML, Lichtenstein P, Lundström S, Larsson H, Micali N, Taylor MJ, Bulik CM. Etiology of the broad avoidant restrictive food intake disorder phenotype in Swedish twins aged 6 to 12 years. JAMA Psychiatry. 2023;80(3):260–9.
8. Mancuso C, Izquierdo A, Slattery M, Becker KR, Plessow F, Thomas JJ, Eddy KT, Lawson EA, Misra M. Changes in appetite-regulating hormones following food intake are associated with changes in reported appetite and a measure of hedonic eating in girls and young women with anorexia nervosa. Psychoneuroendocrinology. 2020;113:104556.

Chapter 2
Psychological Assessment and Treatment

The initial goal of the psychological assessment should be to confirm a diagnosis and ARFID subtype (selective eating, chronic low appetite/interest, or fear of aversive consequences) [1], as well as to ensure that there aren't also concerns for other eating issues. Sometimes, patients will deny body image issues or intentional restriction of food and claim to have early satiety or fear of abdominal discomfort, nausea, or vomiting, but it becomes clear over time that anorexia nervosa is the more appropriate diagnosis. Individuals might resist weight restoration or may only be willing to conduct food exposures with lower calorie food options. The clear presence of intentionally restrictive eating, desire to lose weight, or compulsive exercise makes the diagnosis of anorexia nervosa more likely, although eating disorder experts do also sometimes see patients with longstanding ARFID symptoms who later develop symptoms more consistent with another eating disorder diagnosis.

A comprehensive psychological assessment by a mental health provider is needed to establish an ARFID diagnosis while also screening for the presence of additional mental health conditions that may complicate the picture. Ideally, parents and the individual should participate in the assessment, and it may be necessary to obtain collateral information from other treatment providers, childcare workers, extended family members, and/or teachers for diagnostic clarification.

Typically, it helps to start by making introductions, setting the family at ease, explaining the process for the evaluation so they know what to expect, and building rapport with the child. Clinicians who see patients with ARFID should have child friendly toys and games or paper and crayons for drawing to keep them entertained. Many are much younger than the patient population typically seen in most eating disorders clinics.

There may be some intentional overlap with questions from other providers on the team, but it is important to consider the answers through the lens of a mental health provider. As with any other presenting concern, identify the main problem, and elicit a history of when and how it began. Was the onset abrupt or gradual? Was

A. B. Sinha et al., *Comprehensive Clinical Care for Adolescents with Avoidant/Restrictive Food Intake Disorder (ARFID)*,
https://doi.org/10.1007/978-3-031-92232-9_2

there a clear trigger? How has eating evolved over time? Does anything make it better or worse? Depending on the age of the patient and their comfort, the provider may ask questions directly of the patient, or history might be taken largely from the parent's perspective. Take a 24-h food recall of everything eaten the previous day, including amounts and times if possible. Was this a typical day of eating? Are there any patterns in eating? Any sorts of sensitivity to flavors, smells, textures, noise, or temperature? Are they fearful of something negative happening related to eating, such as pain, nausea, vomiting, or choking? Are there safe foods that the patient is always able to eat? Are there some that they are sometimes able to eat? Do they have "food jags" in which they consume the same item repeatedly for several days or weeks before moving on to another favored item? How does the family handle mealtimes? Does the family eat together, or do individual members grab meals and snacks when schedules permit? Can the patient eat at restaurants or family functions? Do the parents make multiple meals to account for the patient's preferences? Are mealtimes pleasant and light, or marked by irritability, tension, and fighting? Are the patient and parent worried, or are they coming for evaluation at the insistence of a pediatrician or other specialty provider?

Developmental history is often key to sorting through the presenting issue in ARFID. Were there any problems or complications with pregnancy, delivery, or infancy? Did the patient have medical interventions or neonatal or pediatric intensive care unit (NICU/PICU) stays in early life? Did they ever need a feeding tube? Kids with significant medical issues in early life may have ongoing challenges related to feeding due to not being exposed to the mechanics of eating at the normal developmental stage. Some also have chronic sequelae related to medical trauma in early life. Did they meet developmental milestones within the appropriate time frame? Temperamentally, were they a colicky, anxious, or intense baby, or were they more relaxed? Elicit a history of feeding. Were there issues with nursing (troubles latching or low milk production), or did they need to experiment with different formulas for whatever reason? Did they struggle with weight gain or growth? How did the process of introducing new foods go? i.e. At what age did the process begin? Were they excited and curious about new foods, or was it a struggle? Did they prefer liquids to solid foods? Discovering the answers to these questions can also be helpful in identifying the need for early intervention services for speech, physical therapy, or occupational therapy in early life, as this may indicate longer standing concerns about growth and development.

Once a full history of eating issues has been obtained, the clinician should perform a screen of psychiatric review of systems and further flesh out any areas of concern before moving on to the remainder of the diagnostic interview. This includes mood, anxiety, externalizing disorders, autism, psychosis, and obsessive-compulsive spectrum conditions. With any pertinent positives, it will be important for the clinician to tease apart the timeline of symptom development in the context of eating issues. This helps to determine whether mood, anxiety, poor concentration or other symptoms are truly co-occurring conditions as opposed to signs and symptoms of malnutrition.

The remainder of the evaluation includes a thorough exploration of medical history, family medical and psychiatric history, physical review of systems, and social history. The social history is particularly important as it gives insight into the level of difficulty this child is having. Are they attending school and functioning at their baseline, or are they having challenges making/keeping friends, getting into trouble, having behavioral challenges across domains, or failing to attend school or complete their work? Do they have an individual educational plan (IEP) or 504 plan in place to support their academic growth and development? Is the school aware and responsive to concerns? The review of more sensitive identity issues and habits should be completed privately (as developmentally appropriate) with explanations to the parent and patient about the limits to confidentiality. Gender identity can be important if there is body dissatisfaction present that is not related solely to weight and shape concerns. Desire to prevent the development of secondary sex characteristics may impact eating in a variety of ways that are important to understand.

The remainder of the evaluation should include an evaluation of mental status and review of any available survey data (such as the patient health questionnaire [PHQ 9], generalized anxiety disorder [GAD 7], and ask suicide screening questions [ASQ]). Objective medical data (height, weight, vital signs, laboratory data, electrocardiogram) can inform the overall picture but interpretation should be deferred to medically trained clinicians. Additional survey measures can be useful for research purposes or to track progress over time. The ARFID module of the Eating Disorder Evaluation (EDE) [2], the Pica ARFID and Ruination Disorder Interview (PARDI) and Nine Item ARFID Screen (NIAS) are empirically validated measures that can be used in this population. The PARDI is a semi structured interview lasting around 45 min [3], while the NIAS is a short screen [4]. The Food Neophobia Scale (FNS) is a 10-item measure that examines willingness to try new foods but does not help to distinguish subtypes [5].

After gathering all relevant data, the clinician ideally would work with a multidisciplinary team to determine the appropriate treatment plan moving forward. Patients generally benefit from working with a team of clinicians with eating disorder experience who can work together effectively and communicate closely to support them [6]. This often includes a medical provider, a mental health clinician, a dietitian, a psychiatric provider (if needed), and an occupational therapist if OTs with interest and experience are available. In some areas, speech language pathologists (SLP) tend to be involved as opposed to OT. In areas where this expertise is not available, the other members of the team may be able to take on some of the important roles that OT/SLP colleagues play in supporting the ARFID population.

Is the patient medically and psychiatrically stable for outpatient care? If it is safe to proceed with outpatient management, what level of care is most appropriate? Typically, the goal is for children and teens (and even young adults in many cases) to recover at home with the care and support of their families. Historically, many teams used to think that it was ideal to step down through all levels of care to gradually return to outpatient treatment. We now know that this is not necessary and that many families are able to successfully transition from inpatient to outpatient treatment. However, there are some cases that benefit from a more immersive experience with additional structure and support in place. Most treatment centers caring for ARFID patients are more traditional eating disorder programs that offer an ARFID track in addition to more usual programming for anorexia nervosa or bulimia nervosa.

Levels of Care

- Inpatient medical: focused on correcting the sequelae of severe malnutrition; typically, short stays that are determined by achieving weight restoration or correction of vital sign instability or laboratory abnormalities
- Inpatient psychiatry: a locked setting that provides safety and containment for those with active suicidal ideation, non-suicidal self-injury, or other co-morbidities that are preventing the individual from being able to care for themselves in a less restrictive environment.
- Residential treatment center (RTC): mental health treatment programs that provide 24-h supervision and oversight. However, they are not locked units so may not be appropriate for those with acute safety concerns. Programming consists of group, family, and individual therapy along with therapeutic challenge outings.
- Partial hospitalization program (PHP): mental health treatment programs that provide many of the milieu and therapeutic activities that are offered in residential settings. These are programs in which patients return home in the evenings (and often weekends) which allows some additional opportunity to practice managing eating and behaviors in a less restrictive setting.
- Intensive outpatient program (IOP): mental health programs offering afternoon and evening programming. These programs can be attractive to those needing added support while also wanting to remain enrolled in school or actively working. This allows patients to be able to continue to return to their usual life activities in a more gradual and stepped manner [7].

For those who can safely transition to outpatient treatment, the family needs to decide what modality will work best for their needs. The usual evidence-based approaches include family -based treatment and individual cognitive behavioral therapy approaches. Child and adolescent patients participating in cognitive behavioral therapy (CBT) also benefit from the involvement of parents and/or other caregivers in the treatment process.

Family based treatment (FBT) is the approach with the most data to support its use in adolescent anorexia nervosa, but it has been adapted for use in the treatment of other eating disorders, including ARFID [8]. The main tenets of FBT include taking an agnostic approach, parent empowerment, and externalization of the illness. Parents are encouraged to use their experience and knowledge of their child and family to implement strategies to renourish their child, although this may be more challenging in cases of long standing low appetite or selective eating. The treatment approach focuses on being forward thinking and solution focused rather than spending a lot of time speculating on the reasons for the development of disordered eating. This is a manualized protocol consisting of approximately 22 sessions over the course of 6 months, and all family members participate in treatment sessions. In FBT for anorexia nervosa and bulimia nervosa, sessions are broken down into three phases, but this may not be necessary in ARFID if the patient is pre-adolescent [9].

In the first phase of treatment, parents are encouraged to take over planning, purchasing, preparing, and plating all meals and snacks. The patient learns that not eating is not an option, and the parents work to implement structure and support throughout the day to normalize eating patterns and make sure that adequate nutrition is taken in. The second session includes a family meal that allows the therapist to have more insight into the realities of eating in the home. Participation in school, activities, sports, and pleasant events is leveraged to encourage eating. The family generally first works to increase the amount of nutrition taken in, and then works to increase the food repertoire if needed. Parents use their judgment to decide how they would prefer to approach the situation, but the principles of exposure and response prevention are generally very helpful throughout the process. This involves psychoeducation about the anxiety process, followed by learning strategies to manage anxiety, and finally practicing challenging situations in vivo so that the individual can solidify coping skills and strategies. Generally, developing a food hierarchy can be a very effective way to reintroduce fear foods. The family identifies foods that the child would like to be able to eat, then works on ranking them from easiest to most challenging. The family may incorporate strategies of chaining and shaping to help the child gradually expand food choices. For example, the patient may only want to eat one brand of chicken nuggets. The family might first work to incorporate different brands of chicken nuggets, followed by different iterations and/or shapes of breaded chicken (patties, tenders, dinosaur shaped nuggets). They might next choose to work on trying new dipping sauces or sides. Families should remember that it often takes multiple exposures for an individual to truly decide how they feel about a new food.

Patients are ready for phase two of FBT when the patient is in a medically stable place, there is little pushback at mealtimes, and the parents feel confident about allowing the patient some increased independence. Phase two should be a gradual process during which the patient is able to plate meals and snacks under supervision or is allowed to eat lunch independently at school without observation. The frequency of visits should decrease from weekly to biweekly at this time, but parents should be willing and able to jump in to increase observation or support if the child is struggling in any way.

Phase three of FBT is generally shortest, and the transition takes place when the child is able to eat independently. Phase three may not be indicated in pre-adolescent patients. During phase three, meetings occur monthly, and the focus shifts to relapse prevention and discussion of normative developmental challenges that may have been pushed to the back burner while dealing with more acute food related concerns.

Initial pilot studies suggest that FBT-ARFID is more effective than usual medical care, with patients gaining weight throughout treatment. Scores on the PARDI decreased, suggesting a reduction in symptom severity [10]. Additional studies are currently underway.

The number of sessions varies depending on acuity and need. Our experience is that patients with fear of aversive consequences may respond more rapidly to treatment as they generally have a history of normalized eating which provides a template for them to work to get back to. Individuals with the other two subtypes might be more challenging to treat given that they tend to have very long standing and entrenched eating habits. The family may have difficulty appreciating the urgency of the situation or need to make change, and may need a slightly more directive approach to avoid falling back into old habits and patterns.

Cognitive behavioral therapy for ARFID (CBT-AR) is used in patients older than 10 years and is appropriate for each subtype, as long as the patient is medically stable, able to tolerate oral feeds, and is not reliant on enteral feeding. Treatment typically consists of 20–30 sessions over 6–12 months and is split into four stages [11]. Sessions may be individual, or family supported, but the interventions are the same, regardless of the people involved. Individual sessions may be most appropriate for highly motivated, older teens, while younger patients who may be less motivated or need to restore larger amounts of weight often benefit from parental involvement [12]. The first stage of treatment focuses on psychoeducation regarding ARFID and the CBT intervention, while the second stage shifts to education about nutrition and deficiencies. Stage three is the meat of the treatment and uses graduated in session exposures to target maintaining mechanisms. Finally, stage four focuses on relapse prevention and identifies strategies for future practice. As with FBT, CBT-AR has been studied across the lifespan, with very promising results. In one pediatric study, 70% of patients no longer met criteria for ARFID at the end of treatment, and 85% of mental health clinicians rated patients as "much improved" or "very much improved." Underweight patients restored more than 10 pounds, and an average of 17 new foods were incorporated into their diets [13].

Additional interventions such as Supportive Parenting for Anxious Childhood Emotions (SPACE-ARFID), Feelings and Body Investigators—ARFID Division (FBI), and Picky Eaters Clinic focus on younger children [14]. SPACE is a 12 session intervention targeting parental responses to eating behaviors, while Picky Eater's Clinic is a parent only seven session group intervention that helps refine parent management techniques and teaches strategies to expand food variety. FBI is geared toward younger kids [4–10], and provides a playful way to teach interoceptive awareness and gradual exposures to help children and their parents better understand and tolerate physical experiences with eating and anxiety that often lead to food avoidance [15].

More research is needed in order to determine the best psychological approach to ARFID treatment. However, current interventions and studies available suggest that it is important to involve parents in the treatment process, and that the most successful interventions are tailored to focus on the specific needs of the patient and family. This includes ARFID subtype as well as chronological age and developmental stage.

Mental Health Assessment

History of Present Illness

- Timeline of symptom development
- Inciting or triggering event
- Specific challenges with eating
- Weight trends
- 24 h food recall
- Rule out intentional restriction, compulsive exercise, binge-purge behaviors
- Explore presence or absence of features associated with certain ARFID subtypes
  - Selective eating
  - Low appetite/interest
  - Fear of aversive consequences (pain, emetophobia, choking)
- Psychiatric review of systems and safety assessment
  - Mood
  - Anxiety
  - ADHD and externalizing disorders
  - Autism spectrum disorders
  - Psychosis
  - Post-traumatic stress disorder
  - Substance use disorders

Past medical history

- Major medical conditions
- Surgeries
- Injuries

Past psychiatric history

- History of therapy interventions
- Medications prescribed for psychiatric conditions
- Hospitalizations
- Suicide attempts or non-suicidal self-injury

Family medical and psychiatric history

- Medical conditions
- Eating disorders
- Other psychiatric conditions
- Substance use disorders
- History of completed suicide

Social and developmental history

Pregnancy, delivery, developmental milestones
Living situation
Family constellation and relationships
School name and grade
Academic accommodations (IEP, 504, special education)
Typical academic performance
Activities
Peer relationships
Gender identity and sexual orientation
Trauma and abuse
Substance use

Mental Status Examination

References

1. Norris ML, Spettigue W, Hammond NG, Katzman DK, Zucker N, Yelle K, Santos A, Gray M, Obeid N. Building evidence for the use of descriptive subtypes in youth with avoidant/restrictive food intake disorder. Int J Eat Disord. 2018;51(2):170–3. https://doi.org/10.1002/eat.22814.
2. Schmidt R, Kirsten T, Hiemisch A, Kiess W, Hilbert A. Interview-based assessment of avoidant/restrictive food intake disorder (ARFID): a pilot study evaluating an ARFID module for the eating disorder examination. Int J Eat Disord. 2019;52(4):388–97.
3. Bryant-Waugh R, Micali N, Cooke L, Lawson EA, Eddy KT, Thomas JJ. Development of the Pica, ARFID, and rumination disorder interview, a multi-informant, semi-structured interview of feeding disorders across the lifespan: a pilot study for ages 10–22. Int J Eat Disord. 2019;52(4):378–87.
4. Zickgraf HF, Ellis JM. Initial validation of the nine item avoidant/restrictive food intake disorder screen (NIAS): a measure of three restrictive eating patterns. Appetite. 2018;123:32–42.
5. Pliner P, Hobden KL. Development of a scale to measure the trait of food neophobia in humans. Appetite. 1992;19(2):105–20.
6. Brewerton TD, D'Agostino M. Adjunctive use of olanzapine in the treatment of avoidant restrictive food intake disorder in an eating disorders program. J Child Adolesc Psychopharmacol. 2017;27(10):920–2.
7. Derenne J. The role of higher levels of care for eating disorders in youth. Child Adolesc Psychiatr Clin N Am. 2019;28(4):573–82.
8. Lock J, Robinson A, Sadeh-Sharvit S, Rosania K, Osipov L, Kirz N, Derenne J, Utzinger L. Applying family-based treatment (FBT) to three clinical presentations of avoidant/restrictive food intake disorder: similarities and differences from FBT for anorexia nervosa. Int J Eat Disord. 2019;52(4):439–46.
9. Lock JD. Family-based treatment for avoidant/restrictive food intake disorder. New York: Routledge; 2021.
10. Lock J, Sadeh-Sharvit S, L'Insalata A. Feasibility of conducting a randomized clinical trial using family-based treatment for avoidant/restrictive food intake disorder. Int J Eat Disord. 2019;52(6):746–51.

11. Kambanis PE, Thomas JJ. Assessment and treatment of avoidant/restrictive food intake disorder. Curr Psychiatry Rep. 2023;25(2):53–64. https://doi.org/10.1007/s11920-022-01404-6. Epub 2023 Jan 14. PMID: 36640211; PMCID: PMC10211369.
12. Thomas JJ, Eddy KT. Cognitive-behavioral therapy for avoidant/restrictive food intake disorder: children, adolescents, and adults. Cambridge: Cambridge University Press; 2019.
13. Thomas JJ, Becker KR, Kuhnle MC, Jo JH, Hardhman SG, Wons OB, Keshishian AC, Hauser K, Breithaupt L, Liebman RE, Misra M, Wilhelm S, Lawson EA, Eddy KT. Cognitive-behavioral therapy for avoidant/restrictive food intake disorder: feasibility, acceptability, and proof-of-concept for children and adolescents. Int J Eat Disord. 2020;53(10):1636–46.
14. Menzel JE, Perry T. Avoidant restrictive food intake disorder: review and recent advances. Focus. 2024;22:288–300.
15. Zucker NL, LaVia MC, Craske MG, Foukal M, Harris AA, Datta N, Savereide E, Maslow GR. Feeling and body investigators (FBI): ARFID division-an acceptance-based interoceptive exposure treatment for children with ARFID. Int J Eat Disord. 2019;52(4):466–72.

Chapter 3
Psychiatry

The psychiatric care of patients with eating disorders is limited by the fact that there are no medications that have been approved by the Food and Drug Administration (FDA) for the treatment of pediatric eating disorders. There are a limited number of medications with an FDA indication to treat adults with bulimia nervosa [1] and binge eating disorder [2]. Despite the lack of an FDA indication, psychiatric providers working with eating disorders can and do use psychotropic medications off label to target symptoms that are impacting the ability to take in adequate nutrition.

In general, the approach to using medication in eating disorder patients is to use established treatments to target co-occurring disorders that may be impacting nutrition [3]. For example, antidepressant medications may be necessary to treat long-standing mood or anxiety disorders that are present in a patient who also has disordered eating.

Establishing a timeline of symptoms is an essential part of the assessment process when working with patients with eating disorders. Malnutrition can lead to the signs and symptoms typically associated with depression, as well as increased anxiety and difficulties with focus and concentration. It is important to consider symptoms elicited in this context, as adding medication treatments for mood, anxiety, or attention deficit hyperactivity disorder (ADHD) is unlikely to be beneficial (and may even be harmful) if the underlying and unifying cause for the symptoms is better explained by malnutrition [4].

When prescribing medications to patients with malnutrition, it is important to remember that medically compromised patients may be vulnerable to adverse side effects. It often is useful to start at low doses and carefully uptitrate as clinically indicated and tolerated. Providers also must be alert to electrolyte abnormalities that might impact treatment. For example, malnourished patients might have low potassium, phosphate, or magnesium levels that could put them at risk of developing a prolonged QTc interval, which can evolve into a life-threatening arrhythmia known as *torsades des pointes.* Serotonin reuptake inhibitors can also prolong the QTc, as can ondansetron, which is sometimes given to eating disorder patients experiencing nausea. A baseline electrocardiogram (EKG) should be checked and monitored ongoing to be sure that the QTc interval remains in the normal range [5].

A. B. Sinha et al., *Comprehensive Clinical Care for Adolescents with Avoidant/Restrictive Food Intake Disorder (ARFID)*,
https://doi.org/10.1007/978-3-031-92232-9_3

While patients with anorexia nervosa do not seem to benefit from medications known to increase appetite, patients with ARFID do often benefit from appetite promoting agents. Cyproheptadine can stimulate appetite [6] but is also known to have anti-serotonergic properties (which is the reason it is sometimes used to treat serotonin reuptake inhibitor (SSRI) related side effects) so providers need to take that into consideration if using in a patient taking medications for depression or anxiety.

Mirtazapine has been used successfully in a number of ARFID patients owing to its reputation for increasing appetite [7]. There are also some case reports and case series suggesting it reduces nausea and vomiting, improves gastric emptying, and reduces anxiety in this population [8, 9]. The prescribing clinician must weigh the pros and cons of deviating from the gold standard (SSRI or selective norepinephrine reuptake inhibitor [SNRI]) for mood or anxiety treatment in this population. Anecdotally, the SSRIs/SNRIs tend to be better anxiolytics and antidepressants but they take longer to work. Mirtazapine's appetite stimulating and anti-nausea effects anecdotally tend to start to work much sooner and can be used in conjunction with other therapeutic strategies to support renourishment.

Benzodiazepines can be useful to bridge anxiolysis [4] in individuals having difficulty getting fork to mouth, while waiting for more appropriate medication interventions to become effective. The preferred strategy is to use long-acting formulations for short periods of time to minimize the habit-forming potential and decrease the long-term cognitive risks.

The atypical antipsychotics can be very impactful in ARFID treatment, especially in patients with behavioral dysregulation [10, 11]. These medications quickly reduce anxiety, calm irritability, and promote appetite and weight restoration. They are intended to be used in the short term. Baseline laboratory data should be obtained and monitored for any changes consistent with metabolic syndrome [12], although these medications are generally used so briefly that this is not a concern. Often, starting an SSRI shortly after initiation of the atypical is a helpful strategy to optimize anxiety control and prevent long term monotherapy with an atypical. Many ARFID patients end up needing to take anxiolytics in the longer term owing to the high prevalence of co-occurring anxiety in this population, and families can be fearful of making changes to medications once they have experienced some benefit.

The presence of ADHD is often a concern in ARFID patients. Some families find that severe inattention and hyperactivity makes it impossible for the child to sit down and attend to a meal, while others find that stimulant medications can decrease appetite and further hinder efforts to take in adequate nutrition. An astute psychiatric provider can work with the family to better understand the symptoms, and pick and adjust a medication that is least likely to cause side effects. A recent study suggests that most ARFID patients with ADHD are able to continue and adjust their medications without adversely impacting medical stability, which is important as clinicians may be tempted to hold all ADHD medications for fear of worsening appetite [13].

Psychotropic medications can be a useful adjunct in the overall treatment approach to ARFID, particularly when there are co-occurring symptoms like severe anxiety that are impacting renourishment efforts. It is important to establish a clear timeline of symptoms to help determine the presence of true co-morbid diagnoses as opposed to mood and anxiety symptoms that can best be explained by the presence of malnutrition. Prescribing clinicians need to be alert to medical issues that might impact a patient's ability to tolerate psychotropic medications, and need to work collaboratively with other members of the team to best support all clinical interventions.

References

1. Fluoxetine Bulimia Nervosa Collaborative Study Group. Fluoxetine in the treatment of bulimia nervosa. A multicenter, placebo-controlled, double-blind trial. Arch Gen Psychiatry. 1992;49(2):139–47.
2. Hudson JI, McElroy SL, Ferreira Cornwell MC, Radewonuk J, Gasior M. Efficacy of lisdexamfetamine in adults with moderate to severe binge-eating disorder: a randomized clinical trial. JAMA Psychiatry. 2017;74(9):903–10.
3. Ali Z, Couturier J. Psychopharmacology review for eating disorders among children, adolescents, and adults. Focus. 2024;22(3):307–11.
4. Couturier J, Isserlin L, Spettigue W, Norris M. Psychotropic medication for children and adolescents with eating disorders. Child Adolesc Psychiatr Clin N Am. 2019;28(4):583–92.
5. Mehler PS, Watters A, Joiner T, Krantz MJ. What accounts for the high mortality of anorexia nervosa? Int J Eat Disord. 2022;55(5):633–6.
6. Noel RJ. Avoidant restrictive food intake disorder and pediatric feeding disorder: the pediatric gastroenterology perspective. Curr Opin Pediatr. 2023;35(5):566–73.
7. Anttila SA, Leinonen EV. A review of the pharmacological and clinical profile of mirtazapine. CNS Drug Rev. 2001;7:249–64.
8. Gray E, Chen T, Menzel J, Schwartz T, Kaye WH. Mirtazapine and weight gain in avoidant and restrictive food intake disorder. J Am Acad Child Adolesc Psychiatry. 2018;57(4):288–9.
9. Naguy A, Roshdy R, Al-Mutairi A, Alwetayan S, Alamiri B. Mirtazapine improved eating patterns in avoidant/restrictive food intake disorder. Am J Ther. 2023;30(2):173–5.
10. Spettigue W, Norris ML, Santos A, Obeid N. Treatment of children and adolescents with avoidant/restrictive food intake disorder: a case series examining the feasibility of family therapy and adjunctive treatments. J Eat Disord. 2018;6:20.
11. Brewerton TD, D'Agostino M. Adjunctive use of olanzapine in the treatment of avoidant restrictive food intake disorder in an eating disorders program. J Child Adolesc Psychopharmacol. 2017;27(10):920–2.
12. Kameg B, Champion C. Atypical antipsychotics: managing adverse effects. Perspect Psychiatr Care. 2022;58(2):691–5.
13. Finn D, Menzel J, Gray E, et al. Pharmacotherapy for attention deficit/hyperactivity disorder in youth with avoidant restrictive food intake disorder: a case series of patients prescribed stimulant medication in a partial hospitalization program for eating disorders. J Eat Disord. 2023;11:226.

Chapter 4
ARFID: Medical Evaluation and Management

Role of the Medical Clinician

For patients with ARFID, the medical clinician (simplified to "clinician" for the remainder of this chapter) is often the first point of contact for concerned families and/or patients. The clinician's role may include identifying the underlying diagnosis, assessing medical stability, managing the medical sequelae that may be present secondary to malnutrition, and helping to identify the appropriate team members to best achieve stability and recovery.

Evaluation

The initial evaluation of a patient with suspected ARFID should include an assessment of medical stability which can be determined based on a thorough history, physical examination, and pertinent laboratory studies. Based on these findings, appropriate triage can occur (does the patient need to be admitted for medical stabilization?) and additional treatment recommendations can be configured. Because reported behaviors and concerns may vary based on ARFID subtype, it is helpful to be aware of the wide range of possible findings during the assessment process.

History

When obtaining the medical history, it is important to assess weight and growth history, exercise history, and diet history with a particular focus on any past recommendations to alter the diet. It is not unusual for patients to have been recommended

A. B. Sinha et al., *Comprehensive Clinical Care for Adolescents with Avoidant/Restrictive Food Intake Disorder (ARFID)*,
https://doi.org/10.1007/978-3-031-92232-9_4

by health professionals to eliminate specific foods or food groups in hopes of better managing physical symptoms (examples include gluten-free diets, "FODMAP" diets, or specific allergen-free diets). In addition, families may have adopted specific ways of eating due to other family members' needs; for example, gluten-free households due to a sibling's celiac disease or meat-free households due to a family's cultural or religious beliefs.

Unlike in anorexia nervosa, patients with ARFID are not adjusting their eating habits in order to lose weight or change body shape. However, they may disclose avoiding eating or consuming certain foods to avoid abdominal discomfort, nausea, or vomiting. This avoidance can also be reported by patients with anorexia nervosa or other body image-driven disorders and require time and monitoring to discern the primary driver of the eating behaviors.

Past medical and psychiatric history is important, particularly if a patient is more medically complex and has other medical diagnoses that could increase the likelihood of developing ARFID [1, 2]. For example, patients with feeding intolerance due to prematurity, cardiac defects, or GI illnesses may be at greater risk for developing ARFID. Patients with a history of autism spectrum disorder or anxiety may be at increased risk of developing ARFID, as well.

A thorough review of all systems can be useful for both identifying other primary medical concerns, as well as assessing potential medical sequelae due to the underlying malnutrition secondary to ARFID. For example, in a patient with vomiting, it is important to assess for visual changes, headaches, or electrolyte disturbances that could suggest an oncologic process as the source of vomiting. Or, for a patient with low interest/low appetite and chronically low weight, could an underlying systemic illness such as celiac disease or inflammatory bowel disease be the source of malnutrition? With malnutrition, patients may commonly disclose dizziness, fatigue, lightheadedness, stomach fullness and bloating, constipation, decreased concentration, and mood lability.

As opposed to other types of eating disorders, patients with ARFID, particularly the sensory type, are more likely to present with specific vitamin and mineral deficiencies due to narrow food variety. Deficiencies of Vitamin A, C, D, thiamine, folate, and iron should be considered in patients who may have more extreme and specific food avoidance.

Physical Assessment

As part of the physical assessment, vital signs and accurate weight and height should be obtained. Weight and height should be measured with the patient in a gown, having voided prior to the measurement in order to minimize any variation from excess fluid. To determine the degree of malnutrition, one can determine the percentage of median body mass index (mBMI) based on the weight and height [3]. To determine this calculation, one divides the current BMI by the BMI that would place the patient at the 50th percentile for their age on a standard BMI growth chart, multiplied by 100:

$$\text{Percentage mBMI} = \text{Current BMI} / \text{50th percentile BMI} \times 100$$

For example, for a 12 year old female, the 50th percentile BMI, according to the CDC BMI growth chart, would equal about 18 kg/m^2. If her current BMI is 14 kg/m^2, then her percentage mBMI equals 14/18 × 100 or 77.7% mBMI. There are published values for malnutrition that can correspond to the calculated mBMI:

- Mild malnutrition: 80–90% mBMI
- Moderate malnutrition: 70–79% mBMI
- Severe malnutrition: <70% mBMI

In addition, degree of malnutrition can be determined by degree of weight loss or rapidity of weight loss, though both of these determinations require at least two data points to calculate [4].

If growth charts are available, it can be very helpful to look at the overall growth trajectory. Depending on the type of ARFID, different weight and growth histories can be expected:

- Sensory: With this subtype, growth patterns are least predictable as they are highly dependent on the type of foods being consumed. For example, if a patient prefers crunchy, fried textures (such as French fries and chicken nuggets), growth may be at a normal or higher percentile.
- Low interest: It is not unusual to see patients with lifelong trending on a lower percentile growth curves.
- Fear of aversive consequences: Frequently, patients will have a sudden drop-off from their prior growth curve reflecting the decrease in intake associated with the more abrupt development of ARFID.

Recommended vital signs include orthostatic heart rate, orthostatic blood pressure, and temperature. Orthostatic measurements are obtained after a patient has been lying down for 5 min. Then, pulse and blood pressure are measured in the supine position, followed by an upright measurement after the patient has been standing for 2 min.

The physical exam component of the evaluation should include a thorough examination to help support the appropriate primary diagnosis, as well as note other pertinent medical complications. Notable findings can include:

- General: Thin body habitus with appearance of weight loss as noted by muscle wasting, temporal wasting, loss of subcutaneous tissue
- Skin: Presence of lanugo, dry skin and brittle nails, orange discoloration to the skin (hypercarotenemia)
- Head/Neck Throat: Parotid fullness or enamel erosion with frequent vomiting
- Cardiovascular: Slow heart rate
- Gastrointenstinal: Abdominal fullness and tenderness associated with impaired gastric motility and constipation

- Extremities: cool hands and feet that may be pale or blue-ish in color due to poor perfusion (acrocyanosis)
- Neurological: May appear cognitively slower with poor memory or focus

Laboratory and Diagnostic Studies

Given that many of the reported ARFID symptoms (such as fullness, low appetite, nausea) have an overlap with other illnesses or diseases, it can be challenging to determine how much screening to include in an initial evaluation. Often, clinicians may start with more general screening laboratory work. As with any medical diagnoses, if a patient does not respond to treatment in an expected manner or follow an expected timeline, it is prudent to re-assess and explore additional medical explanations.

The initial laboratory evaluation should screen for possible primary issues contributing to the symptoms, as well as screen for medical complications resulting from malnutrition [5].

Initial screening for primary etiologies may include:

- Complete blood count (CBC)
- Complete metabolic profile
- Thyroid studies (TSH, free T4, total T3)
- Erythrocyte sedimentation rate (ESR)

Initial screening for medical sequelae may include:

- Vitamin D level (25-OH Vitamin D)
- Sex hormone levels (such as estradiol, testosterone, follicle stimulating hormone (FSH), and luteininzing hormone (LH))
- Liver function tests (AST and ALT)
- May consider additional vitamin and mineral levels (ferritin, folate, Vitamin B12, zinc) depending on the clinical presentation.

Similar to laboratory studies, other diagnostic studies are ordered based on the clinical concerns of each patient. An EKG is frequently obtained as it can assess for any conduction abnormalities that may be present due to malnutrition. Bradycardia and prolonged QTc interval are two of the more common EKG findings in malnutrition. If a patient is taking any medication that might prolong the QTc (such as antiemetics or anxiolytics), an EKG is even more important to obtain.

Additional studies will be more targeted. For individuals with concern for growth stunting, a bone age can assess their current growth compared to normative values, as well as be used to predict their ongoing growth potential. Measurement of bone mineral density can be considered if there are concerns of stress fractures or low bone mineral density due to prolonged amenorrhea; guidelines typically indicate a lack of menses for 6 months or more as a reason to consider a bone dual energy x-ray absorptiometry (DXA) study [6].

When Do I Admit to the Hospital?

After conducting the initial history and physical exam, the clinician needs to determine if a patient is medically safe to be managed in the outpatient setting or requires an inpatient medical admission. Multiple societies have published recommendations for when to consider admission based on vital signs, weight, and electrolyte levels [4, 7–9]. Findings that might indicate need for admission include:

- Bradycardia: Heart rate of less than 50 beat per minute during the day
- Hypotension: Blood pressure of less than 90/45 mmHg in adolescents, less than 90/60 mmHg in adults
- Orthostasis by pulse: Change in pulse of more than 40 beats per minute in adolescents, more than 30 beats per minute in adults, when moving from a supine to standing position
- Orthostasis by blood pressure: Drop in systolic blood pressure of more than 20 mmHg in both adolescents and adults when moving from a supine to a standing position
- BMI: Less than 75% median BMI in children and adolescents, BMI less than 15 kg/m^2 in adults.
- EKG abnormalities (such as prolonged QTc)
- Electrolyte disturbances

In addition, more specific concerns such as syncope, dehydration, or uncontrollable vomiting might necessitate an inpatient admission for further evaluation and stabilization. As different subtypes of ARFID may present in different ways, it is helpful to consider the medical complications that might be most relevant for an individual:

- Sensory: Depending on the nature of the sensory issue, weight may or may not be a concern for these patients. However, ensuring appropriate micronutrient and macronutrient levels is critical as they can become markedly disrupted if the dietary intake is very narrow in scope.
- Low interest: As many of these patients have had more chronic eating concerns, they may not have the vital sign instability that is typically associated with malnutrition. Often, they are admitted based on low body weight—a calculation that can be challenging to determine when their growth curves may have been chronically low. However, with the increased metabolic needs associated with adolescent growth, the stable-low growth curves may become even lower during this time and warrant additional support.
- Fear of aversive consequences: As many of these patients often present with more abrupt changes in intake, they are often at higher risk of medical instability due to severe malnutrition and weight loss. A close assessment of vital signs is essential.

Medical Management

Once a diagnosis has been determined and medical complications identified, the clinician needs to determine the management plan. Typically, management of patients with ARFID can benefit from a multidisciplinary team, though the exact make-up of that team may vary based on the specific needs of the patient (please see Chap. 7 for additional details on creating a multidisciplinary team). The clinician's role includes stabilizing any medical complications, as well supporting the establishment or return to more appropriate eating behaviors.

As with other eating disorders, stabilization of vital signs relies on improving and sustaining appropriate nutrition. This is typically achieved through a meal plan that will provide the estimated calories, as well as the micro- and macro-nutrients, that are needed. While oral feeding is preferred, nasogastric tube feedings can be needed during specific situations if oral feeding cannot be established in a timely fashion (please see Chap. 9 for more information on nasogastric tube considerations).

When considering the feeding plan, a clinician must help determine the weight gain goals which are often, but not always, necessary. Weight goals are determined by assessing the previous growth history and setting the target to previously tracked percentiles. However, with ARFID, previously tracked percentiles, in both weight and heights, may be significantly lower due to lifelong eating and feeding difficulties [10]. In those cases, clinicians often revert to using a BMI goal along the 10th percentile, though more evidence-based recommendations are needed for this population. If weight gain is necessary, many programs will use a rate gain goal of between 3 and 5 pounds per week in the inpatient setting and 1 and 2 pounds per week in the outpatient setting. It is important to note that for the fear of aversive consequences subtype, initial weight gain may be slower compared to the other subtypes. As the underlying fears are addressed and previous eating patterns re-established, weight gain rates improve.

While establishing the feeding plan, clinicians can provide symptomatic support that may alleviate some of the discomfort associated with the renourishment phase. Gastrointestinal symptoms, such as bloating and constipation, are not uncommon and are due to delayed gastric motility from malnutrition. During this period before motility improves, clinicians can consider medications such as polyethylene glycol, which is typically well tolerated, to manage constipation. Bloating may respond to simethicone or warm packs applied to the abdomen. Pro-motility agents are typically avoided as they may have side effects and/or interactions with other medications commonly used in this population.

While the nutrition plan is being implemented, clinicians should be aware of the risk of refeeding syndrome for patients who may be increasing their intake from a period of restrictive eating [10–13]. Patients with a greater degrees of malnutrition (based on percentage of mBMI or degree of weight lost) are at increased risk, and refeeding syndrome is typically considered more for those patients requiring hospital admission due to their higher level of medical instability. With the introduction of higher calories, patients may be at risk for electrolyte derangements, particularly phosphorus, magnesium, and potassium. To prevent refeeding syndrome, meal plans should be advanced thoughtfully and with close monitoring (daily) of electrolyte levels for at least the first several days.

Once a patient no longer requires an inpatient setting or if they are stable to be monitored in an ambulatory setting, consistent medical follow-up is helpful to ensure any medical complications are resolving and nutritional goals are being met. Depending on the patient needs and the presence of other team members, frequency of medical visits could occur from weekly to monthly intervals. Once nutritional and medical progress is being made, medical visits can decrease in frequency.

Conclusion

The medical evaluation of patients with ARFID is an important piece to ensuring appropriate medical diagnoses are made and medical complications are managed. Though most patients can be successfully managed in the outpatient setting, some patients will require an inpatient medical admission to ensure their stabilization and safe renourishment. Being aware of expected and potential medical complications will support the recovery process whether in the inpatient or ambulatory setting.

References

1. Katzman DK, Norris ML, Zucker N. Avoidant restrictive food intake disorder. Psychiatr Clin North Am. 2019;42(1):45–57.
2. Zimmerman J, Fisher M. Avoidant/restrictive food intake disorder (ARFID). Curr Probl Pediatr Adolesc Health Care. 2017;47(4):95–103.
3. Golden NH, Jacobson MS, Sterling WM, et al. Treatment goal weight in adolescents with anorexia nervosa: use of BMI percentiles. Int J Eating Disord. 2008;41(4):301–6.
4. Society for Adolescent Health and Medicine. Medical management of restrictive eating disorders in adolescents and young adults. J Adolesc Health. 2022;71:648–54.
5. Mehler PS, Andersen AE. Eating disorders: a comprehensive guide to medical care and complications. 4th ed. Baltimore: Johns Hopkins University Press; 2022. p. 237–58.
6. Misra M, Golden NH, Katzman DK. State of the art systematic review of bone disease in anorexia nervosa. Int J Eat Disord. 2016;49(3):276–92.
7. Academy for Eating Disorders Medical Care Standards Committee. Eating disorders: a guide to medical care. 4th ed. Reston: Academy for Eating Disorders; 2021.
8. Crone C, Fochtmann LJ, Attia E, et al. The American Psychiatric Association practice guidelines for the treatment of patients with eating disorders. Am J Psychiatry. 2023;180(2):167–71.
9. Hornberger LL, Lane MA, Committee on Adolescence. Identification and management of eating disorders in children and adolescents. Pediatrics. 2021;147(1):e2020040279. https://doi.org/10.1542/peds.2020-040279.
10. Downey AE, Richards A, Tanner AB. Linear growth in young people with restrictive eating disorders: "inching" toward consensus. Front Psych. 2023;14:1094222.

11. Khan LU, Ahmed J, Khan S, et al. Refeeding syndrome: a literature review. Gastroenterol Res Pract. 2011;2011:410971.
12. Mehler PS, Winkelman AB, Andersen DM, et al. Nutritional rehabilitation: practical guidelines for refeeding the anorectic patient. J Nutr Metab. 2010;2010:625782.
13. Garber AK, Sawyer SM, Golden NH, et al. A systematic review of approaches to refeeding in patients with anorexia nervosa. Int J Eat Disord. 2016;49:293–310.

Chapter 5
Nutrition

Introduction

Registered dietitian nutritionists (RDN) play a tremendous role in helping patients of all ages who struggle with eating disorders and disordered eating patterns. It is customary for hospitals to implement a systematic nutrition risk screening tool to detect patients at risk for malnutrition [1]. All ARFID patients have eating challenges and will be deemed at nutritional risk, thus alerting the clinical dietitian to perform a detailed nutrition assessment and treatment plan. With adequate nutrition care that addresses the patient's immediate nutrition needs, the quality of life and overall health of the patient will improve, and consequently reduce medical costs and decrease length-of-stay [2].

Given that it is also a restrictive eating disorder, those with ARFID may experience similar symptoms and malnutrition complications as those with anorexia nervosa (AN). However, standardized inpatient protocols or outpatient approaches for treatment of AN are likely not the most appropriate treatment approach for those with ARFID. Clinicians and researchers now know that individualized behavioral treatment plans and strategies are often needed [3–5]. Close nutrition management is imperative not just for acute nutrition rehabilitation but for creating long-term behavioral changes. Close collaboration with patients and their caregivers, as well as meal planning, have been incredibly beneficial in addressing this eating disorder. Each ARFID patient has their own unique challenges and the multidisciplinary team will help problem solve and come up with creative solutions to address the individual's and family's needs [6–9].

A. B. Sinha et al., *Comprehensive Clinical Care for Adolescents with Avoidant/Restrictive Food Intake Disorder (ARFID)*,
https://doi.org/10.1007/978-3-031-92232-9_5

Initial Nutrition Assessment

Before meeting a patient and family, it can be helpful for the RD to first consult with any other team members about the patient's presentation and situation. Knowing some background information can help identify the type of nutrition intervention and resources/handouts needed. For example, an inpatient with ARFID sensory subtype will likely benefit from an individualized meal plan, necessitating additional time during the initial sessions to plan and then inform ancillary hospital staff.

When meeting a patient and family for the first time, take the time to provide a full introduction of the dietitian's role. Oftentimes, patients and families report feeling misunderstood by past dietitians or other providers that may have been too prescriptive or generalizing with their recommendations. A thorough introduction can help set expectations, decrease anxiety, and create a safe, trusted space where the patient and family can feel more comfortable honestly answering nutrition-related questions during the session.

The introduction can include answering the following questions:

1. What is a dietitian?

   A dietitian is a core member of the treatment team and will assess the patient's nutritional needs, develop a nutrition plan and provide education on how to best meet those needs.
2. What is your personal experience working with ARFID?

   If you have limited experience with ARFID, you can name that and state that you are actively learning more about it. More importantly, you understand how imperative it is to individualize care according to the patient's and family's needs and, therefore, will be closely collaborating with them and the team.
3. What does the clinical nutrition assessment include?

   The assessment will include, but is not limited to, weight history, growth charts, lifelong diet history and food preferences, physical activity, medical history, and their current medical and eating presentation.
4. How often is the nutrition follow-up and future RD involvement?

   During an inpatient stay, the RD may need to briefly check in daily to execute successful individualized meal planning but usually the RD provides twice weekly follow-up visits. ARFID patients' nutritional plans tend to be dynamic and may require different approaches. Therefore, daily communication with the team, ancillary staff, and the patient and family may be essential in providing an effective and clear plan. In outpatient levels of care, the RD can best determine the frequency of follow-up depending on the patient's and family's needs.

A standard nutrition assessment can be performed as usual, but the following questions and recommendations can be very helpful in understanding the nuances with which an ARFID patient can present:

- 24 h diet recall:
  - Choose a day that is recent
  - Is this a typical day or not? If not, why?

  - Obtain specifics (i.e. brand names of foods, eating setting, portion amounts, condiments used)
  - Any beverages consumed?
  - Any food eaten outside of meals and snacks?
  - Include a caregiver or a close support person (e.g. sibling, friend, etc) in the conversation

- Food allergies, sensitivities, intolerances:

  - What are the symptoms?
  - What age was this discovered? What led to the discovery?
  - Is there a family history of allergies or intolerances?
  - Have formal allergy tests been conducted?

- Nutrition history and current nutrition approach:

  - Is there a specific diet, meal plan, or nutrition approach that is being followed? Was this suggested by another clinician?
  - Frequency and duration of meals/snacks? Any differences between weekdays vs weekends?
  - Has eating changed over time? If so, how?
  - Eating setting (i.e. dining table, bedroom, in the car, school, restaurant, friend's house)?
  - Currently, what are the favorite and most disliked foods?
  - When was the last time a new or unfamiliar food was introduced and/or consumed?

    Is there any avoidance based on the smell, texture, taste, or appearance of the food?
  - Are there any vitamin, mineral, or other nutrition supplements being taken?
  - Are there any currently or previously used formula supplements or modulars (specialized single or multiple nutritional components designed to be added to enhance the nutritional value of one's diet) [10]
  - Is there any history of tube feeds?
  - In general, what is the diet or nutrition approach for the rest of the family?
  - How does the family respond to and accommodate the patient's food preferences?
  - What are the easiest and hardest meals to eat? To prepare?
  - Which meal is the most interesting to eat?
  - When is the patient the most hungry and most full?
  - When is the latest and earliest time to eat?
  - What are the dynamics of the household? Who is involved in meal preparation, plating, and purchasing?
  - Are there any financial constraints? Food insecurity?
  - How does culture play a part? Any cultural practices or differences?
  - Has the family noticed any peculiarities when the patient is drinking or eating (i.e. assessment of oral motor skills)?

The family can be especially helpful in answering these questions since some patients may forget their nutrition history and historical food preferences or may not be as detailed. We've heard some caregivers say:

- "He used to eat everything but is now afraid to eat anything that is not labeled."
- "She's always been a picky eater, even as a baby! She had such a hard time transitioning from the bottle to solid foods and she would spit out most foods I gave her except for cereal."
- "Because she is allergic to peanuts, we don't typically have a lot of nuts at home but now she's scared of any cross contamination and is only eating fruits, vegetables, and meat."

After the initial nutrition assessment has been completed, the dietitian will make a recommendation for the best nutrition approach to follow. In an inpatient unit, the meal plan will need to be carefully planned and discussed with the multidisciplinary team, ancillary staff, and the patient and family.

It can be helpful to mention to the patient that the nutrition approach can always be modified over time, and the patient and family will be collaborative members of the nutrition planning process. Explicitly saying this usually helps decrease any trepidation and can provide reassurance that their individual nutrition needs and preferences will be closely considered. This can help build rapport and initiate a trusting relationship, which will be paramount in creating successful nutrition interventions.

Nutrition Approach at a General Pediatric Unit

On a general hospital floor, the patient will have more autonomy and less structure with the nutrition approach. Typically, patients will be given a general menu and will be expected to choose what, when, and how much to eat. A more hands-on approach, guided by the dietitian, is strongly recommended as it is more efficient to help address malnutrition, incorporate specific food preferences, and increase the overall caloric intake. The dietitian can advise on how much to order, what food and beverage combinations should be selected, which foods to focus eating on, which foods to try, or what nutritional supplements should be included.

Nutrition Approach at a Specialized Inpatient Eating Disorder Unit

Compared to those admitted on a general pediatric unit, the nutrition management of a patient admitted to a specialized inpatient eating disorder unit is usually much more involved. Upon admission, patients are generally started on a set menu with established entrees, side items, and snacks distinguished by prescribed daily calories [11]. For instance, there is a set menu for an 1800 calorie diet vs. a 2400 calorie diet. For some ARFID patients, deviating from the standard protocol of a set menu may be more appropriate. In that case, the patient will get to choose what they want for meals and snacks and the nursing staff may be asked to document what the patient has consumed. Patients are typically encouraged to follow a nutrition plan with three meals, two snacks per day. All patients receive meals/snacks at the same time since there is a set schedule for the kitchen and milieu. Following a consistent meal and snack schedule can help the body adjust to the frequency of eating, regulate hunger and satiety cues, and allow engagement in therapeutic groups and activities. Meals are encouraged to be eaten within 30 minutes and snacks within 15 minutes. If a meal or snack replacement* is needed, the patient is given another 10 min to finish the replacement (*will discuss in the next section titled "Replacement"). A patient may be given extra time to complete their nutrition if that is part of their individualized treatment plan set by the treatment team.

Meal Planning

Inpatient Care

Upon admission, the treatment team can consider prescribing a meal plan that either provides a similar caloric amount the patient was typically consuming prior to admission or one that is higher. Research has shown that patients starting on a higher calorie meal plan (2000 kcal) is safe [11, 12]. However, starting at baseline can also help avoid overwhelming the patient.

A starting lower caloric meal plan may be in the 1000–1400 calorie range. Meals will typically have one to three different food items presented, and snacks consist of one item. Initiating a higher calorie meal plan may start around 2000 calories. Meals may have four or five different food items presented, and snacks generally consist of two items.

Examples of Caloric Breakdowns of Meals/Snacks per Calorie Prescription

1,000 calories/day	
Breakfast	300 calories
Lunch	300 calories
Afternoon snack	50 calories
Dinner	300 calories
Evening snack	50 calories

1,400 calories/day	
Breakfast	400 calories
Lunch	400 calories
Afternoon snack	100 calories
Dinner	400 calories
Evening snack	100 calories

2,000 calories/day	
Breakfast	400 calories
Lunch	500 calories
Afternoon snack	300 calories
Dinner	500 calories
Evening snack	300 calories

2,800 calories/day	
Breakfast	600 calories
Lunch	800 calories
Afternoon snack	300 calories
Dinner	800 calories
Evening snack	300 calories

3,500 calories/day	
Breakfast	800 calories
Lunch	900 calories
Afternoon snack	450 calories
Dinner	900 calories
Evening snack	450 calories

The main specifics of the patient's prescribed meal plan will include the calorie prescription, a list of foods provided at every meal and snack, and portion amounts.

It's especially helpful to establish a patient's nutritional baseline by documenting what and how much of the food has been consumed during the first day(s) of admission. If the patient was able to select choices on a menu, the dietitian should keep track of what was chosen and why. Most hospitals have an order for a calorie count available, which can help the dietitian collect this data. A calorie count is a written log that lists everything the patient has consumed (i.e. food or beverages provided by the hospital, food or beverages from outside of the hospital, condiments, dietary supplements), typically recorded by a nurse or nursing assistant.

Especially at the beginning of the admission, the meal plan presented to an ARFID patient should primarily consist of foods they are currently willing to eat. On occasion, they can also be presented with foods they previously consumed but stopped eating due to their ARFID issue. Provision of familiar, preferred foods can help ease the patient into the nutrition plan and quickly build success in correcting malnutrition, addressing nutrition compliance, and achieving weight restoration [9]. Throughout the admission, food exposures (i.e. new foods, challenging foods, etc.) may be part of the nutrition plan, and may be approached in a similar fashion as Food Chaining. Food Chaining is a method where one can expand their food repertoire by providing new or different foods that share similar characteristics as one's currently consumed foods [13].

Lower Levels of Care

In partial hospitalization programs (PHP) or intensive outpatient programs (IOP), the RD can use a 24 Hour Diet Recall to get a rough idea of the patient's baseline intake [14]. From there, a recommendation to increase the energy amount can be prescribed and gradual inclusion of other foods can be recommended over time. Micronutrient deficiencies can also be investigated and addressed. Active collaboration and a more directive approach with the patient and family will be key in seeing success in increased energy and variety of intake while in the program and at home.

In the outpatient setting, follow-up care may not be as frequent and therefore focusing on realistic, tangible goals is the best approach. Keep in mind that the patient and family may have approached nutrition in a particular way for several years, and thus, may require a lot of time and psychoeducation to help create seismic nutritional shifts in the patient's eating. Starting with one to three goals to help build small successes can be a great jumpstart. Also, a detailed sample meal plan with different calorie prescriptions can be a helpful guide to follow at home (see page ___ in the Appendix for a sample meal plan). However, it is advisable to caution caregivers about the implications of knowing and emphasizing calorie amounts of food items and how it can lead to disordered eating practices or can unintentionally undermine the actual nutritional value of the food. Therefore, it would be best to speak of calories in a more neutral way such as reframing it as "energy" or specifying the macro- or micro- nutritional benefits of the food item instead.

The 5 Food Guide©

The 5 Food Guide© and The 5 Food Basic Guide© (a more simplified version) were created by this dietitian, Allyson Sy, MS, RD to serve as a tool to learn about the patient's food preferences (see Chap. 22, Appendix 1 and Appendix 2). As early as possible during an inpatient admission or in the course of an outpatient nutrition assessment, the dietitian can ask the patient and/or caregiver to complete this list because it will serve as the ultimate guide to individualized meal planning.

This list includes most commonly eaten foods and beverages, categorized by meal/snack and food group. The patient should use a marker or highlighter to color code every food on the list based on the degree of interest in and familiarity with the food according to the assigned colors:

- Red - dis liked foods; not currently eaten
- Yellow - neutral foods; sometimes eaten
- Green - most loved foods; currently eaten
- Blue - previously eaten foods; not currently eaten
- Purple - new or unfamiliar foods that can be tried

The 5 Food Guide© can be used differently depending on the patient presentation or ARFID subtype. For the lifelong sensory eater, it can be helpful to also ask their parents to fill it out since parents typically remember their child's blue foods the best. For the fearful eater, the main focus will be on the foods they *c*urrently feel safe eating (indicated in green) and the previously eaten foods (indicated in blue). Within the list of blue foods, it's important to ask the fearful eater what foods they'd feel most comfortable reintroducing again. It's helpful to have parents separately fill out the list as well since parents tend to best remember what the patient used to eat comfortably before the fear started to impact their eating. The RD can then cross reference both 5 Food Guides© to create the most appropriate nutrition plan that incorporates currently and previously preferred foods.

In addition to the patient's food preferences, additional factors to consider when meal planning include:

- Volume—consider what is realistic and manageable for the patient at that time
- Variety—consider inclusion of hospital, home, or outside restaurant foods
- Energy density
- Prioritization of specific macronutrients and micronutrients
- Inclusion of all or most food groups
- Consider amount of liquids vs solids
- Cohesion—make sure the meal makes sense and appears appetizing
- Different textures, which can help gather more information about the patient's feeding patterns
- Familiarity—easy to eat foods (preferred foods) vs. new or challenging foods
- Is this economically, culturally, and religiously appropriate for the patient and family?
- Plate Model guidelines or other nutrition framework to be followed that can then be taught to the patient and family

The Plate Model for Recovery: "Picture the Plate©"

Introducing the framework of how meals will be ideally constructed can be described by referring to the plate model for recovery, "Picture the Plate©" [Fig. 5.1] (see Chap. 22, Appendix 3). No matter what meal plan the patient starts on, "Picture the Plate©" can be a great visual guide on how to best put together a nutritionally balanced meal for their recovery, and beyond. This approach intentionally moves away from specifying numbers and helps move towards the concepts of intuitive eating by relying more on visual cues.

"Picture the Plate©" depicts an image of a standard dinner plate divided into the main 5 food groups: grains/starches, fruits and vegetables, dairy/dairy alternatives, fats, and protein. Seeing the plate divided in such a way can be a great, simplistic tool for someone to take note of what a nutritionally balanced meal can look like.

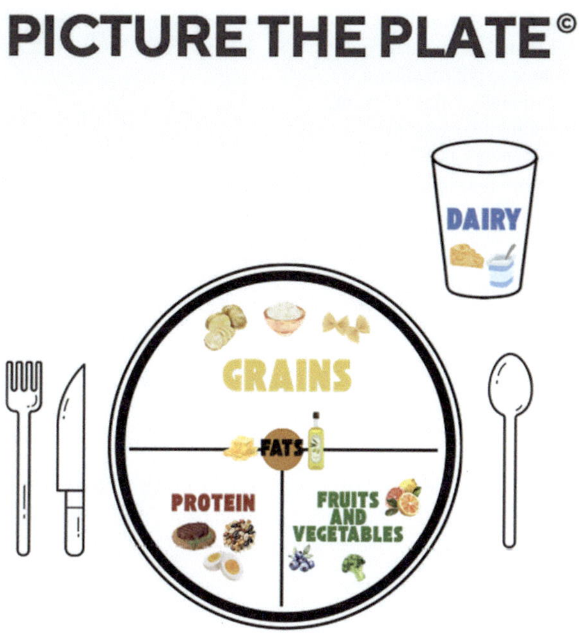

Fig. 5.1 Picture the Plate, A visual guide of how to put together a nutritionally balanced meal for individuals who: have a history of malnutrition, have high energy needs, are on weight restoration plan, who are very physically active or who need a catch-up growth plan

Patients that have a history of malnutrition, have high energy needs, are on a weight restoration plan, are very physically active, or need to exhibit catch-up growth can benefit from "Picture the Plate©", which emphasizes the importance of grains/starches making up the bulk of the meal (50% of the plate). Starches will provide the malnourished body with the glucose and energy that it needs to meet the high energy demands during nutrition rehabilitation. Protein will help build and repair muscle. Fruits and vegetables provide water, fiber, and micronutrients to correct nutrient deficiencies and promote regularity. Dairy provides adequate calcium and vitamin D to promote bone density. Fats promote brain development, organ protection, and a surge of calories when used in small portion amounts [15].

For other patients that have lower energy needs, may not need to be weight restored, or are more nutritionally and medically stable with low to moderate physical activity, there is a different version of a plate model for recovery. "Picture the One Third Plate©" [Fig. 5.2] depicts a meal that has a more equalized distribution of the grains/starches, protein, and fruits and vegetables food groups (see Chap. 22, Appendix 4). These meals include more fruits and vegetables and protein and less grains, which ultimately can provide less calories.

In the beginning, if possible, the dietitian should aim to provide at least three different food groups per meal with the goal to eventually include all of the five food groups. The patient and family will benefit from continued nutrition education about "Picture the Plate©" or meal plan so they can continue to follow this approach at home and beyond.

In regards to snacks, using a standard snack plate for visualization can be helpful, however, snack items greatly vary in size, portion, and amounts. There is no

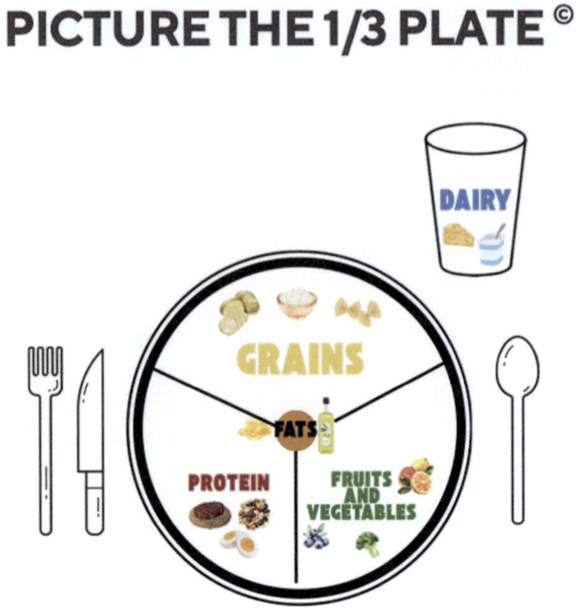

Fig. 5.2 "Picture the 1/3 Plate", is a visual guide on how to put together a nutritionally balanced meal for individuals that have lower energy needs, may not need to be weight restored, or are more nutritionally and medically stable with low to moderate physical activity

standard visualization but there can be a recommendation to emphasize plating more energy dense foods or providing more foods within the grains, protein, fats, or dairy food groups.

For more detailed information about the plate model for eating disorder recovery, The Plate-by-Plate Approach® is another version that is thoroughly explained in *How to Nourish Your Child Through an Eating Disorder* and *How to Nourish Yourself Through an Eating Disorder*, which are great resources for patients, families, and providers [16].

Meal/Snack Replacement Approach: The Eat-Replace Model

As briefly mentioned earlier, nutrition replacement can be provided if the patient is unable to consume everything expected at a meal or snack. The replacement type will be chosen based on what the patient likes and tolerates the best. The amount of replacement necessary will first be determined by the treatment team. In the inpatient setting, replacement is typically offered and encouraged to be consumed orally but if the patient is unable to do so, it can be administered enterally [17].

Adequate intake is imperative and replacement plans help emphasize the importance of taking in an appropriate amount of nutrition. Patients can practice eating the recommended amount with a back-up plan in place all while the stomach gets acclimated to the expanding volume. For example, if the patient consumes everything except for the half bag of chips on their lunch plate, then the replacement provided can be of equivalent caloric value so the patient can remain 100% meal plan compliant and meet their estimated energy needs.

In lower levels of care and/or at home, replacement doesn't have to be of the same caloric value as the foods not consumed. Replacement can be offered in small portioned or full bottle amounts for ease of calculation and distribution. For instance, an entire meal can be equivalent to 2 bottles of a 1.5 kcal/mL nutritional formula (total of ~700 calories) and if a patient is able to eat at least 50% of the meal but is unable to finish 100% of it, then the replacement can be 1 bottle. If the patient eats less than 50% of the meal, then the replacement can be 2 bottles. Another option would be to think of the replacement in 25% increments, especially if the patient is still adjusting to volume. If the patient doesn't finish the entire meal but eats at least 75% of it, replacement can be ¼ of a bottle.

Replacement is intended to be a "quick fix" so choosing a replacement in the form of a liquid nutritional supplement (e.g. Boost Plus, Ensure Plus, Boost VHC, Lutrish, or similar formula is ideal. To help minimize volume, choosing the best tolerated energy dense supplement allows them to fully complete the replacement in a relatively short period of time (10 min or less) as well as allow adequate digestion and development of hunger for the next meal or snack. If a patient is unable to tolerate a liquid replacement, the team can consider using an energy dense food replacement (e.g. energy bars, nut butter sandwiches, cookies, nuts, etc.) instead. However, this may require more chewing and digesting, and thus, more time to complete. It may also lead to burnout. Other replacement options to consider include homemade energy dense smoothies, milkshakes, or energy dense retail liquid supplements.

The team can always modify the approach to build the ability to tolerate the eat-replace model. At each meal or snack, the patient can consume a specific amount of replacement, no matter how much of the meal/snack was completed. It is best to start off with a very small amount so that the patient can successfully finish (e.g. 1 oz. Boost Plus or 6 whole almonds). Over time, the team can either continue to prescribe increasing amounts of replacement to finish at every meal or snack or proceed with the standard protocol of the "eat-replace model" (i.e. the replacement provided is only calorically equivalent to the food not consumed at the meal/snack).

Trouble Shooting the Eat and Replace Model:

Patient Is Able to Drink Replacement with No Issues

- Recommend the best supplement for the patient and consider the following factors when making a decision: taste, texture, caloric density, ease of purchase or availability, cost, nutrient content, and age appropriateness
- Families appreciate supplements that are economical and easy to purchase.

Patient Dislikes the Taste of Most Supplements, Especially Those that Come in "Milky" Chocolate, Vanilla, or Strawberry Flavors

- Consider a formula that has a fruit juice flavor (such as apple, citrus, berry).

Patient Is Able to Drink a Limited Volume of Replacement

- Work to gradually increase the volume of the supplement and consider making the supplement more caloric.
- Consider energy dense formulas currently available on the market (ie Lutrish, Boost VHC, Ensure Compact)
- Consider modifying the formula to be more energy dense: add ice cream, nut butters, chocolate syrup, oil, heavy whipping cream, coconut milk, etc. Can use modulars or food enhancers such as Duocal, Beneprotein, ProMod, Microlipids. Since the overarching nutrition goal is to get the patient to eat solid food, including real food is always a preferred strategy.
- If the patient is really volume limited or timid about the eat and replace model, OT and RD can first specify a minimal amount of replacement that is mandatory to consume at every meal and snack while the patient is getting used to this model and while the patient is getting used to eating a certain amount of food again.
- Example Meal Plan of 1000 calories/day with Specified Supplementation Needed:

  Breakfast: 300 calories +60 ml Ensure Plus
  Lunch: 300 calories +60 ml Ensure Plus
  Afternoon Snack: 50 calories +30 ml Ensure Plus
  Dinner: 300 calories +60 ml Ensure Plus
  Evening Snack: 50 calories +30 ml Ensure Plus

    60 ml Ensure Plus = 2 oz. = ~90 calories
    30 ml Ensure Plus = 1 oz. = ~45 calories

This meal plan provides a certain amount of food based on the calorie distribution. The patient can eat however much they want of that food. Whatever food is leftover, they do not have to drink the replacement for. Instead, they must always consume their specified amount of supplementation.

However, if the patient is able to finish 100% of the food, then they do not need to consume the replacement.

Patient Prefers Something Other than Nutritional Formula Supplements

- Find retail beverages that are as calorically dense as possible
- Most retail beverages are not as calorie dense and require a lot more volume than the standard nutrition supplements. Simply showing the volume differences to the patient can help them better understand why nutrition supplements are the preferred beverage choice at this point.

Patient Is Unable to Tolerate a Liquid Supplement

- Choose an energy dense food replacement from the patient's list of "safe" foods [Table 5.1].
- The patient should enjoy or easily tolerate eating the chosen food for replacement. However, they may become tired of this food so it's still important for the patient to push through exposures or the meal/snack served.

Once the meal plan and replacement plan are established, the nutrition plan gradually evolves in overall volume, calories, variety, and complexity.

Table 5.1 Examples of energy dense foods for replacement

Nut butter and Jelly Sandwich, Grilled cheese sandwich	Peanut butter filled pretzels, chocolate covered pretzels
Protein bars, Granola bars, Nut bars	Peanut butter cracker sandwiches, Cheese cracker sandwiches
Cookies, Biscuits, Baked goods (i.e. croissants, pound cake, etc.)	Nuts, Seeds
Chips, Crackers	Trail mix
Ice cream, Ice cream sandwiches Frozen nutrition supplement formulas (to resemble ice cream)	Bagels, Garlic bread
Cheese	Pudding, Nutrition supplement puddings
Chocolate	Chocolate covered nuts, Chocolate covered dried fruit

The treatment team will be working diligently to help challenge the patient enough to make strides towards recovery but not too much that it leads to many failed attempts. Extreme frustration can lead to setbacks and difficulties trusting the care team.

Creating a Meal Plan with Exposure Foods

When starting food exploration/expansion, start by asking the patient some of these questions:

- Are there some foods that your friends eat that you wish you could eat?
- Are you able to eat at your friend's house for birthdays, sleepovers, etc.? If yes, how so? If not, what would you like to be able to eat when there?
- Is there anything at home that smells good or that you wish you could eat?
- Are there any upcoming field trips, parties or events that you plan on going to?

  What would you need to be able to eat so that you can easily go to these functions and not have to plan or worry so much about your nutrition?

- What are the restaurants that your family goes to regularly? Are there any restaurants that you wish you could eat at?
- For the family:

  What are some of the food staples or foods that you have regularly so that your child is able to eat with you (aka safe/preferred foods)? What are the food staples or food that you have regularly that you wish your child could eat?

Then with the patient: Which of these foods would you like to try?

After gathering information, the dietitian can provide education around the nutritional benefits of foods that are available everywhere or why specific foods would add some nutrient value to the patient's life. For example if they can only eat one brand-specific passion fruit yogurt, expanding to more readily accessible yogurt types could be very helpful. If they do not eat any vegetables, consider starting with a vegetable that is normally available at their house (and, preferably, at restaurants).

Next, start to make a list of potential foods. Together with the patient and parents, decide which food they would like to try first (this may coincide with the "purple" foods on The 5 Food Guide©). If they have any interest in dips or spices, or even if they don't, it can still be helpful, to have sauces/dips ready (e.g., ranch, a preferred salad dressing if they have one, honey mustard, ketchup, hot sauce, oil & vinegar, etc.) and any seasoning that they like at home (e.g. can be cultural spices such as tajin, pepper flakes, cumin, etc.). Adding lemon may also change the flavor of a food. Access to a "changeover" food or drink can also be helpful. A "changeover" food is a highly preferred food or drink they can use to change the flavor in their mouth if they eat something they really don't like.

Once a list of exposure foods has been made, the RD will incorporate them into the meal planning process.

Tips:

- Provide exposure foods that make sense and are easy to add. Especially at the start of this process, set them up for success so the patient can build on that confidence and continue the positive momentum.
- If the patient anticipates the exposure food to be really difficult or is anxiety provoking, the rest of the meal can consist of just their favorite foods, or provide a complementary "changeover" food so that the patient can feel less stressed about the exposure.
- Plan for an exposure food to be the only sweet or dessert food present during a meal. The patient may be more motivated to try it. If a meal already includes a preferred sweet food or dessert, the patient may be less interested in trying the exposure food.

How Much of the Exposure Food Should Be Provided?

Even though exposure foods are less likely to be eaten, provide a standard portion. Or at minimum, provide a smaller sized standard portion, but make sure it is not too miniscule. A standard portion of nuts, for example, is one ounce. For the exposure, a little less than an ounce (i.e a very small handful) can be provided. Do not provide just one nut (unless agreed upon by the treatment team). Providing just one nut may be too limiting, especially if the patient discovers that they like it and wants to actually eat more. However, if the patient eats just one nut from the small handful, that is okay. Having the patient visually see the standard amount can help teach them what a normally eaten amount looks like. Additionally, a patient may discover that they only like certain parts of the exposure food item and can therefore benefit from a bigger portion of it. For instance, if the exposure food were peanut butter filled pretzels and the patient only liked the pretzel part, they may want more pieces of it. Therefore, providing at least two handfuls of these pretzels can be an appropriate amount for the exposure.

Approach to Food Exposures

- Create a list of foods that the patient wants to prioritize and start with their preferred food exposures.
- Involve the patient in the process of planning the food and the exposure including, but not limited to, choosing the variation of that food, the brand, the portion, the meal/snack time, etc.
- Describe what to expect when eating the food (clinician can comment on the taste, texture, smell, etc.).
- Ask the patient to set a goal or an intention when eating the food (does the patient expect to take one bite? Eat the whole portion?)
- Keep track of the foods eaten by having the patient fill out a worksheet titled "The Trial Tracker©" (see handout Appendix 5 in the Nutrition Appendix). This document can help the patient be more aware of how their experiences with food exposures can change over time.
- Typically, it is best to recommend the patient to try at least three bites of the exposure food (any sized bite is fine).

Nutrition Plan of Care Considerations Based on ARFID Subtype

ARFID Subtype: Sensory

Nutrition Plan

- Have the patient complete The 5 Food Guide©. Once completed, implement an individualized meal plan that provides majority preferred foods (green) with some neutral foods (yellow). Try to provide as much variety as possible within this list. The RD ideally should select meal/snack choices to prevent food jags and ensure appropriate caloric intake.
- It may be helpful to ask caregivers to also fill out The 5 Food Guide© based on what they think the patient's food preferences are. Sometimes the patient forgets the previously eaten foods (blue) and caregivers most often always remember what these are. If the caregivers can identify such foods, it would be helpful to eventually introduce these foods again as well.
- Identify the most liked and tolerated nutritional formula and implement the Eat and Replace Model. Choose a replacement plan that best fits the needs of the patient.
- Collaborate with the patient and incorporate challenge and exposure food items. Have the patient complete the Trial Tracker© worksheet to help the patient try

exposure foods in a structured fashion at the start of the meal or snack while recording their progress.

- Provide points and rewards when trying exposure foods to incentivize the patient (i.e. behavior modification plan).
- Sensory eaters dislike unexpected consistency, which is why most have issues with fruit and vegetables. Multiple textured foods (like lasagna) or foods that require excessive chewing (like steak) can also be hard. Work with the patient to figure out the best balance between challenging them with different food textures during a meal or snack.
- Consider serving smaller portions of preferred foods to be plated at a meal so the patient is more inclined to eat the challenge/exposure food. Can also consider serving the challenge/exposure food separately and at the start of the meal when the patient is most hungry. Once the patient is able to eat most (or all) of the challenge food, then serve the rest of the food (which will likely be preferred, easier to eat foods). Through this approach, the patient can have an additional incentive to eat the challenge food first. However, the eventual goal is to have it all on the same plate, served at the same time.

Inpatient Considerations

- Upon admission, can initially start on ad lib PO (patient chooses what to eat and decides how much to eat) with a calorie count.
- Have the patient complete The 5 Food Guide© and then implement an individualized meal plan. Can allow foods from outside and continue to encourage hospital foods as much as possible.
- Test out multiple formula supplements along with different flavors within the first couple days of admission. The patient can use The Trial Tracker© while taste testing. Based on the patient's response and tolerance, proceed with the standard approach of The Eat and Replace Model or prescribe a specific quantity to consume at each meal and snack.
- It can be helpful to collaborate with the patient (and other multidisciplinary team members) almost daily to plan when and how to incorporate challenge/exposure food items.
- Keeping a record of the prescribed meal plans can be helpful for the family to have a copy of upon discharge so they can see how the nutrition plan has evolved over time.

ARFID Subtype: Low Interest

Nutrition Plan

- Have the patient complete The 5 Food Guide©. Once completed, implement an individualized meal plan that provides majority preferred foods (green) with some neutral foods (yellow). Try to provide as much variety as possible within this list. The RD can suggest selecting some meal/snack choices to prevent food jags and ensure appropriate caloric intake but ultimately the meal plan should comprise of foods the low interest eater would be the most willing to eat, especially when prioritizing weight repletion.

- To help build success at the start of the process, consider prescribing a lower calorie meal plan or one that is close to the patient's caloric baseline.
- Implement The Eat and Replace Model with the patient's most liked replacement (liquid or food).
- Ideally apply Picture the Plate© and aim to have as many different food groups as possible, however, if the patient is more motivated to eat certain food groups, can allow this to help meet their energy needs (i.e. a meal may be able to only provide 3 food groups as opposed to the ideal 5).
- Provide energy dense and easy-to-eat foods to help the patient eat within the timeframe or before boredom/reluctance/disengagement ensues.
- Can consider a behavioral modification plan to help incentivize the patient to consume the appropriate nutrition.
- Tips:
  - At home, have the patient be involved in the food preparation process.
  - Play games or provide fun worksheets around eating to make meals more enjoyable (e.g. have them be a "scientist" or food taster/investigator).
  - Choosing the right types of food to provide may be more difficult since the patient's food preferences may change depending on how they're feeling at that moment. They may also be unable to explain why. For example, the patient may not want to eat their favorite entree even if they've been successfully eating it in the past. Thus, this patient may need to rely on replacement more often. If this is the case, can consider providing the option for food trade-in options instead of liquid nutritional formula. Replacement may also include a few options to help increase variety and prevent food burnout (e.g. for one patient, food trade-in options included a PB&J sandwich, milkshake, or ice cream).

Inpatient Considerations

- Use the standard set menu type of meal plan with the standard replacement protocol (see page __, section *Nutrition Approach at a Specialized Inpatient Eating Disorder Unit* for more details).
- Consider allowing trade-ins of foods to help promote food PO intake. For example, if the patient has tried to eat everything but struggles with the french fries because they got too cold or weren't reheated to their liking, allow the patient to swap for a different food (of similar nutritional value) instead of giving replacement. Trading-in of foods should be monitored and discussed with the caregivers and/or treatment team so the patient doesn't negatively take advantage of this accommodation. Constant trade-ins of foods may not always be feasible, can lead to a lot of food waste, can burn out the caregiver (they become a "short order cook"), and can contribute to food avoidance or the facade that the patient should only eat foods they like/can eat all the time.

- Can introduce the eat and replace model standard protocol upon admission, as it allows for the most efficient way to achieve weight restoration and medical stability. This can help expedite the process in which the RD and OT can strategize on how to successfully implement this into the daily meal plan in the hospital and at home. If the patient attempts to consume the replacement but cannot fully finish it, this should be carefully documented so the treatment team is aware of the total caloric consumption. If the patient dislikes the standard formula and/or standard protocol approach, can taste test and consider other replacement options.

ARFID Subtype: Fear of Aversive Consequences

Nutrition Plan

- Ask the patient what their "safe" foods currently are. Can ask the patient to fill out The 5 Food Guide© to better identify their "safe" foods being in green and previously eaten foods in blue. Also ask their caregivers to fill out The 5 Food Guide© based on what the patient used to be able to eat and prefer, before the fear around eating happened since sometimes the patient can't remember their previously eaten foods (blue).
- Prescribe an individualized meal plan that eventually incorporates challenge/exposure foods (ones they used to love and only agree to try).
- Meal Planning Tips:
  - Provide ~75–90% of green foods to help the patient accomplish eating most of the meal. This approach will help the patient feel safe, relaxed, and gain confidence over time.
  - Depending on OT input as well, can provide ~10–25% of the blue foods. Such foods may need replacement if not completely eaten OR these can be plated but NOT need replacement if not completely eaten.
  - It can be helpful including the most aromatic "safe" or previously eaten foods at meals as the patient will have a higher likelihood of eating those foods by simply stimulating their olfactory senses and digestive processes. For instance, smelling french fries from the patient's favorite fast food chain can trigger some positive memories associated with that food and help the body initiate hunger cues.
- Provide a back-up nutrition plan such as the standard approach of "The Eat and Replace Model" or a prescribed quantity of replacement at each eating opportunity.
- Can use a behavioral modification plan or Ladder Block Plan to help with motivation and tracking (see Chap. 9: Behavioral Modification for more details). (Can utilize a template such as BMod Plan Example 1, Appendix 6).
- NOTE: If the patient has had this fear for a longer period of time, has been untreated, and the restricting/limiting of foods have worsened over time, they may likely need a longer term replacement plan and/or long-term treatment.

Inpatient Considerations

- Start with ad lib PO (patient chooses what to eat and decides how much to eat) with a calorie count.
- Trial a small quantity of replacement and use The Trial Tracker© worksheet to rank taste. This helps to neutralize the experience and e considered.

Other Care Considerations

Dealing with Nausea

- Implement OT techniques; consider use of a relief band and/or aromatherapy.
- Explore how to make eating more enjoyable.
- In the beginning of treatment, avoid foods that lead to nausea. Consider smaller meals and snacks and gradually increase volume.
- Some patients have more issues with nausea in the morning or late at night. Consider splitting the breakfast nutrition into a smaller breakfast meal and then a morning snack to make it more manageable. One can also consider providing a smaller evening snack and a bigger afternoon snack.
- Some patients benefit from having access to crackers, nuts, or other preferred foods that they can eat upon waking if they wake up nauseous.
- For medically unstable patients with severe nausea and limited ability to eat, the team may initially need to provide tube feeds to help meet the nutrition needs. This can be traumatic, so should be avoided unless medically necessary.

Dealing with Vomiting

- It is imperative to stop the cycle of vomiting so the multidisciplinary team, patient, and family should collaborate on how to best stop this.
- Provide fewer liquids and foods that are more energy dense (similar to those that are volume restricted or have nausea). Liquids and solids may need to be separated for a period of time if the vomiting is consistent or if the patient does not have control over it.

Dealing with Social Anxiety

- Start with one-to-one meals then work up to family meals at home, then going out to restaurants with family, and then eating with people they are comfortable with (relatives vs friends).
- Once the patient is able to eat with others, first start with snacks and then eventually work up to doing meals together. It may help to predetermine what the patient will eat before going to the restaurant to decrease anxiety about the food. It may also help to tell their friends and family about the child's situation so they can provide a more conducive environment while eating. Discuss options to make the meal supportive such as playing games at the table, listening to music, etc.

Meal Support

- Most ARFID patients benefit from having support while eating a meal or snack, especially during a food exposure. Some tips to consider when providing meal support:
- Discuss exposure food ahead of time and outline goals for that meal or snack ("Let's have you try at least one bite of every food on the plate" or "Let's aim to have you eat 50% of this food")
- When providing an exposure food, there should be familiar preferred foods on the table (e.g. fruit snacks, yogurt, mac and cheese, etc.)
- Provide reminders to take bites, bigger bites, keep eating, etc.
- Utilize distraction tools (music, pleasant conversation, games, trivia)
- Encourage the patient to use coping skills such as deep breaths, grounding, or a tool to help initiate a cold sensation (e.g. a frozen lemon, cold pack, splashing cold water onto the face—TIPP skill used in Dialectical Behavior Therapy [DBT])
- Show or point to the amount of food that needs to be eaten or prioritized
- Ask the patient if they want to start the meal or snack with the new food first or the familiar food first
- Use a timer for accountability if that is helpful
- Provide reassurance and remind the patient that their body can handle and digest the food
- Review their treatment goals
- Normalize that the body may strongly react to a new food but with more bites and exposures, the reaction will get less intense and they may discover that they actually like the food
- Use a worksheet or have the patient journal to reflect and document their eating experience with the new, reintroduced, or non-preferred food

Nutrition Education and Planning

Providing nutrition education along with a sample meal plan can be very helpful.

Unlike for other eating disorder patients and families, creating a menu (including portions and calories listed) may be helpful to get the patient and family started with the amount needed at home. A week's menu that shows a gradual increase in calories and portions can be beneficial and easier to follow along, which an outpatient team can follow up on and keep building from.

For patients who are volume restricted, fruits and vegetables can be served in very small quantities as the other food groups (this food group is lower in calories, can take a lot of time to chew and digest, can take up a lot of space on the plate; for fruits/vegetables with high fiber content, these can also keep the body feeling fuller longer and can worsen constipation). Provide more energy dense foods (e.g. lasagna vs. plain pasta with ground meat) and include different sources of fats into every food presented on the plate. Offer more energy dense liquids at each meal and snack such as milk, juice, smoothies, or milkshakes since these beverages can pack in a lot of nutrition and calories. Provide dessert with lunch and dinner meals, and if feasible, include restaurant food as it tends to be more energy dense than home cooked meals or hospital meals [18]

For the Neurodivergent Eater

- Some find it helpful to have a "body double" or "accountability buddy" so that the patient can follow through on their nutritional goals or tasks. For example, they can designate someone to go grocery shopping with them or ask a family member to stay on the phone as they finish their replacement.
- Consistency and structure are key. They can benefit from set meal/snack times and build a routine that can be successfully followed.
- Consider providing a concrete nutrition plan that may need to specify exact portions or calories—everything can be spelled out if needed.
- It's important to keep the environment supportive and encouraging—not shaming or judgmental.
- Consider flexibility or creativity during challenging situations so that the patient can be successful in completing their overall nutrition.
- Consider simplicity—provide a specific daily meal plan that specifies the foods needed per meal or snack; can consider a varied rotation of meals or snacks which can help limit grocery shopping (but remind the patient of potential for food burnout). As long as the overall meal plan is nutritionally complete, those with neurodivergence are less likely to experience food burnout.
- A behavioral modification plan can also be helpful by listing out self-care goals in addition to nutrition goals (see Chap. 9: Behavioral Modification for more details). (Can utilize a template such as BMod Plan Example 2, Appendix 7).

For the Independent Eater

While family support is strongly recommended, there are instances where an adolescent or young adult may require additional training to support their nutrition, especially if they are living independently (e.g. college, study abroad, etc.). There are also cases where, despite the patient's young age, the parent is not actively involved in their meals and the child is expected to be fully responsible for themselves (e.g. parent(s) are working when the child is at home or child is living in a group home setting), necessitating further training for the patient to manage their nutrition.

- Set alarms to stay on schedule for meals/snacks. This can be incredibly helpful since hunger cues may be minimal or absent. Patients can also get easily distracted or want to avoid eating.
- Keep preferred, shelf-stable foods readily accessible. Advise the patient to always have energy bars, liquid supplements, and dense snacks (e.g. keeping a snack in their backpack/purse, storing a cooler in the car, having food in their

desk drawer, having a snack assortment on the bedside table, etc.) so food is easily accessible wherever they are.

- Have a set rotation of items or a menu for ease.This can be helpful since the patient and/or family doesn't always have to plan the meals or keep thinking about the nutrition plan. This can help set a routine.
- Plan social outings that involve eating. Social meals can allow patients the opportunity to have company while eating, promote enjoyment and social engagement around food, help provide modeling, and can help the patient stay accountable with their meal plan. Additionally, dining out usually means higher calorie foods. Encourage the patient to order dessert, beverages, appetizers to share, etc. However, caution the patient about getting too distracted by table conversations and discuss a plan and tools for the patient to remain engaged with eating no matter the circumstance. Help the patient plan what to order ahead of time and caution the patient when sharing food with others as this may lead to undereating.
- Utilize food delivery services (e.g. take out, already prepared and packaged meals, or groceries) as cooking or preparing meals can be too overwhelming or time consuming.
- Utilize disposable plates and utensils for minimal clean up (for a more sustainable option: purchase biodegradable products) or encourage the use of a dishwasher. Sometimes the idea of cleaning dishes and kitchenware can be a deterrent to food preparation.
- Label food to designate what should be eaten during a meal or snack (or can task someone else to do it). If the fridge or cupboard already has a designated breakfast, lunch, dinner for the day then the patient can easily grab the meal and get it ready for consumption. Having snack bags with perfectly portioned snack items can also be helpful and if using shelf-stable foods, these can be prepared ahead of time and designate the day of the week that it should be consumed.
- Buying groceries in bulk, especially single portioned foods, can help for better tracking of their intake. They can better count calories, have enough food readily available, and minimize grocery shopping.
- Taking medications or multivitamins during a meal or snack can be helpful so two important things can be accomplished at the same time. For some medications or vitamin/mineral supplements, this can lead to better tolerance, absorption, and digestion. Using a pillbox or packing the medication with the meal or snack bag can be helpful in promoting med compliance.
- Identify preferred, "go-to" meals and snacks when the patient is experiencing more challenging situations (e.g. times of illness, low mood or no mood/motivation to eat, when traveling, times of stress or business, etc). It's understandably hard to think about food sometimes when the patient is distracted or emotionally and mentally invested in other things. Caution the patient about food burnout—favorite foods can be helpful during difficult times, but ideally should not be eaten repeatedly.

Family Meal Sessions with an RD

Inpatient and Outpatient Considerations

- Family meals are an opportune time to observe the interactions between family members and the child or teen during a time of eating. A meal, instead of a snack, should be observed. Ideally, this Family Meal should mimic the home environment and what would normally happen during a meal. Advise parents to provide their typical meal, dine where they usually eat, and proceed to act as they normally would. By observing a family meal, the clinician can identify issues that arise while eating and can be addressed as soon as possible.
- The family meal can last around 45 min (30 min for the meal duration; 15 min to debrief).
- If possible, the RD can join the family meal so they can also observe and ask questions that are likely relevant for the other team members to know. The RD can also observe the food and amounts being served.
- Some questions to ask the family: Who decided on what to have for this meal? How was this decided and why? How is this meal different from more typical meals at home? How is it the same?
- What to look out for: topics of conversation, body language between all family members, how the patient handles and interacts with food, table behaviors (e.g. microbiting, eating one food at a time, delay to start), patterns around eating (e.g. only eating white foods first). How does the meal end (do parents stop eating? Does the patient keep eating until the end of time? Does the patient stop eating when they start feeling full or tired?) Was there negotiating or allowance to swap items? Who in the family finished the meal first, and last? How did the parent respond when the patient did not want to eat something or showed anxiety/fear around the food? Was replacement offered and/or provided?
- The family meal can be a time of observation and questioning. During a more private session between the caregivers and/or patient and the dietitian, the RD can provide concrete examples and recommendations to the family that can best help the patient with nutrition support [19]. For instance, the dietitian can help answer the following questions: What could the parent have said instead? When should the parent allow food swaps? How could the patient have eaten more efficiently?
- For future family meals: ask families to provide specific foods (e.g. preferred and non-preferred foods; challenge/exposure foods).

References

1. Reber E, Gomes F, Vasiloglou MF, Schuetz P, Stanga Z. Nutritional risk screening and assessment. J Clin Med. 2019;8(7):1065. https://doi.org/10.3390/jcm8071065.
2. Lin JA, Jhe G, Vitagliano JA, Milliren CE, Spigel R, Woods ER, Forman SF, Richmond TK. The association of Malnutrition, illness duration, and pre-morbid weight status with anxiety and

depression symptoms in adolescents and young adults with restrictive eating disorders: a cross-sectional study. J Eat Disord. 2021;9(1):60. https://doi.org/10.1186/s40337-021-00415-7.
3. Guss CE, Richmond TK, Forman S. A survey of physician practices on the inpatient medical stabilization of patients with avoidant/restrictive food intake disorder. J Eat Disord. 2018;6:22. https://doi.org/10.1186/s40337-018-0212-4.
4. Gorrell S, Vendlinski SS, Thompson AS, et al. Modification of an inpatient medical management protocol for pediatric avoidant/restrictive food intake disorder: improving the standard of care. J Eat Disord. 2023;11:165. https://doi.org/10.1186/s40337-023-00895-9.
5. Tsang KK, Hayes LC, Bujoreanu S, Samsel CB, Ibeziako PI. Characterization study of patients presenting to an acute care pediatric hospital identified with avoidant/restrictive food intake disorder. Hosp Pediatr. 2020;10(7):600–7. https://doi.org/10.1542/hpeds.2020-0010.
6. Eddy KT, Harshman SG, Becker KR, Bern E, Bryant-Waugh R, Hilbert A, Katzman DK, Lawson EA, Manzo LD, Menzel J, Micali N, Ornstein R, Sally S, Serinsky SP, Sharp W, Stubbs K, Walsh BT, Zickgraf H, Zucker N, Thomas JJ. Radcliffe ARFID workgroup: toward operationalization of research diagnostic criteria and directions for the field. Int J Eat Disord. 2019;52(4):361–6. https://doi.org/10.1002/eat.23042.
7. Norris ML, Obeid N, Santos A, Valois DD, Isserlin L, Feder S, Spettigue W. Treatment needs and rates of mental health comorbidity in adolescent patients with ARFID. Front Psych. 2021;12:680298. https://doi.org/10.3389/fpsyt.2021.680298.
8. Sharp WG, Volkert VM, Scahill L, McCracken CE, McElhanon B. A systematic review and meta-analysis of intensive multidisciplinary intervention for pediatric feeding disorders: how standard is the standard of care? J Pediatr. 2017;181:116–124.e4. https://doi.org/10.1016/j.jpeds.2016.10.002.
9. Mairs R, Nicholls D. Assessment and treatment of eating disorders in children and adolescents. Arch Dis Child. 2016;101(12):1168–75. https://doi.org/10.1136/archdischild-2015-309481.
10. Davis A, Baker S. The use of modular nutrients in pediatrics. JPEN J Parenter Enteral Nutr. 1996;20(3):228–36. https://doi.org/10.1177/0148607196020003228.
11. Garber AK, Cheng J, Accurso EC, Adams SH, Buckelew SM, Kapphahn CJ, Kreiter A, Le Grange D, Machen VI, Moscicki AB, Sy A, Wilson L, Golden NH. Short-term outcomes of the study of refeeding to optimize inpatient gains for patients with anorexia nervosa: a multicenter randomized clinical trial. JAMA Pediatr. 2021;175(1):19–27. https://doi.org/10.1001/jamapediatrics.2020.3359.
12. Golden NH, Cheng J, Kapphahn CJ, Buckelew SM, Machen VI, Kreiter A, Accurso EC, Adams SH, Le Grange D, Moscicki AB, Sy AF, Wilson L, Garber AK. Higher-calorie refeeding in anorexia nervosa: 1-year outcomes from a randomized controlled trial. Pediatrics. 2021;147(4):e2020037135. https://doi.org/10.1542/peds.2020-037135.
13. Fraker C, Fishbein M, Walbert L, Cox S. Food chaining: the proven 6-step plan to stop picky eating, solve feeding problems, and expand your child's diet. Volume 1. Boston, MA, USA: Da Capo Press; 2007.
14. Feillet F, Bocquet A, Briend A, Chouraqui JP, Darmaun D, Frelut ML, Girardet JP, Guimber D, Hankard R, Lapillonne A, Peretti N, Rozé JC, Simeoni U, Turck D, Dupont C, Comité de nutrition de la Société française de pédiatrie (CNSFP). Nutritional risks of ARFID (avoidant restrictive food intake disorders) and related behavior. Archives de Pediatrie: Organe Officiel de la Societe Francaise de Pediatrie. 2019;26(7):437–41. https://doi.org/10.1016/j.arcped.2019.08.005.
15. Kiani AK, Dhuli K, Donato K, Aquilanti B, Velluti V, Matera G, Iaconelli A, Connelly ST, Bellinato F, Gisondi P, Bertelli M. Main nutritional deficiencies. J Prev Med Hyg. 2022;63(2 Suppl 3):E93–E101. https://doi.org/10.15167/2421-4248/jpmh2022.63.2S3.2752.
16. Sterling W, Crosbie C, Shaw N, Martin S. The use of the plate-by-plate approach for adolescents undergoing family-based treatment. J Acad Nutr Diet. 2019;119(7):1075–84. https://doi.org/10.1016/j.jand.2018.06.011.

17. Białek-Dratwa A, Szymańska D, Grajek M, Krupa-Kotara K, Szczepańska E, Kowalski O. ARFID-strategies for dietary Management in Children. Nutrients. 2022;14(9):1739. https://doi.org/10.3390/nu14091739.
18. Hornberger LL, Lane MA, Committee on Adolescence. Identification and Management of Eating Disorders in children and adolescents. Pediatrics. 2021;147(1):e2020040279. https://doi.org/10.1542/peds.2020-040279.
19. Lian B, Forsberg SE, Fitzpatrick KK. Adolescent anorexia: guiding principles and skills for the dietetic support of family-based treatment. J Acad Nutr Diet. 2019;119(1):17–25. https://doi.org/10.1016/j.jand.2017.09.003.

Chapter 6
Occupational Therapy Foundation for ARFID: Theory and Frameworks

What Is Occupational Therapy and Why Do Occupational Therapists Treat Patients with Avoidant Restrictive Food Intake Disorder?

Occupational therapy is a health science profession with a background in physiology and mental health [1]. Occupational therapists are dedicated to helping individuals reach their highest functional level. They are trained to provide "activity analysis" in order to examine where an individual has obstacles to reaching their full potential [2]. These barriers could be physical (e.g., a patient with a neurological disorder who cannot walk and eat per their prior baseline), psychological (e.g., a fear of vomiting) or related to organization (e.g., a young adult with ARFID who cannot figure out how to fit 3 meals and 2 snacks into their day). Regardless of cause, occupational therapists are focused on assisting a patient reach their highest functional level with the greatest independence level possible [3, 4]. Occupational therapy addresses a range of interconnected domains and elements to support individuals' engagement in meaningful activities [5]. This approach ensures a comprehensive and personalized intervention strategy.

The following areas are examined for ARFID patients.

The Importance of Occupational Therapy in ARFID Treatment

This section provides an in-depth theoretical base of occupational therapists' work with ARFID patients. Given that many sites do not have an inpatient occupational therapist, this section offers background information for these sites to consider

A. B. Sinha et al., *Comprehensive Clinical Care for Adolescents with Avoidant/Restrictive Food Intake Disorder (ARFID)*,
https://doi.org/10.1007/978-3-031-92232-9_6

including an occupational therapist as part of their team. It also serves as a guide for occupational therapists to use as a foundation for treatment. With their background in physiology and mental health, occupational therapists are especially well-positioned to serve this population [6].

(i) **Occupations (e.g., activities of daily living, rest and sleep, work and education)**

"Occupations" are meaningful activities that individuals participate in within their families and communities. These activities encompass both responsibilities and desired activities [7]. Often, ARFID patients' primary roles include being a student, sibling, child, friend, and sometimes an employee.

Occupational therapists who treat ARFID patients examine the patient's daily living patterns to identify any barriers to adequate and varied nutrition or to living a full, healthy, happy life. For instance, if a patient spends most of their time playing video games and refuses to come for meals, their occupation as a "video game player" disrupts essential daily activities like eating and using the bathroom, which are necessary for health. Similarly, students or employees might struggle with getting up early enough to eat breakfast or with finding time to eat in a school environment. In such cases, their role as a student impacts their feeding activity, which can, in turn, affect their performance. Addressing these issues is crucial for the patient to make behavioral changes and improve their intake, overall health, and outlook. It is essential to examine a patient's activities of daily living and typical schedule to understand and address their barriers to receiving full nutrition at regular intervals.

(ii) **Contexts (Environmental and Personal Factors)**

The environment can significantly influence an individual's ability to obtain adequate nutrition. Firstly, it is important to establish that there are no food insecurity issues. There are times where fiscally a family cannot afford food and this must be addressed [8]. There are also times where there may be food insecurity issues because the patient wants school lunch, but the school lunch lines are too long, the cafeteria food runs out or the patient is not getting sufficient nutrition through their available school-provided lunch. Many patients with ARFID require more than the 30 minutes allocated at lunch to get enough nutrition. Some students may only achieve adequate nutrition if permitted to eat during class, necessitating accommodations from the school. They must feel comfortable eating in class and have access to non-messy food that allows them to continue their schoolwork uninterrupted.

During the COVID-19 isolation period, some ARFID patients improved with constant access to their home fridge, while others struggled more at home [9].The pandemic highlighted the importance of socialization, with documented increases in mental health issues, underscoring its vital role in overall well-being [10].

Environmental factors can impact patients with ARFID, particularly those with Sensory Processing Disorder, Autism, or Anxiety [11]. Eating in a noisy cafeteria or crowded setting can pose significant challenges. Changes in familiar foods or daily schedules can also be distressing, and sensory sensitivities such as cafeteria smells or sounds of chewing can make eating difficult.

(iii) **Performance Patterns (i.e., Habits, Routines, Roles, and Rituals)**

It is well-documented that periods of change or transition, such as starting a new school year or transitioning to summer, can disrupt established behavior patterns [12]. Establishing habits or linking tasks together increases the likelihood of consistent behavior (e.g., taking medication with the same meal daily).

Examining a patient's and their family's eating habits and routines is crucial. For example, if an occupational therapist is working on expanding a patient's food choices but selects a food that no one else in the family eats, the utility of this expansion may be limited due to lower likelihood of purchase or consumption by others. Choosing a food regularly consumed by family members ensures accessibility. If a hospitalized patient is encouraged to adopt a meal schedule (e.g., dinner at 5:30 p.m., snack at 8:30 p.m.), but their family typically dines later, it is crucial to assist the family in incorporating necessary meal intervals into their routine, possibly adjusting the order to better fit their lifestyle.

Family dynamics sometimes involve a desire for adolescents to take on more independent roles in meal preparation and consumption, even if the teen is not yet capable of this level of responsibility. Occupational therapists can assist by gradually building independence skills while educating parents about the patient's current capabilities. This approach might involve starting with supervised independence during certain meal intervals (e.g., snacks) and progressing as appropriate.

Effective routines can positively impact nutritional intake; for instance, ensuring food availability during long commutes to school or activities can increase daily nutrition. Implementing such routines requires thorough activity analysis and planning involving both the patient and their caregivers.

Rituals surrounding food consumption can either facilitate or hinder eating habits. For example, a patient accustomed to a specific snack daily may struggle if it becomes unavailable during travel. Conversely, rituals like having an after-school snack can provide a predictable opportunity for nutritional intake. Patients with Autism Spectrum Disorder (ASD) or sensory issues may have specific rituals related to food packaging or accompaniments (e.g., dips) that, if disrupted, can affect their ability to eat.

(iv) **Performance Skills (i.e., Motor Skills, Process Skills, and Social Interaction Skills)**

Occupational therapists examine a patient's performance skills to understand their impact on the patient's overall functioning [13]. For individuals with ARFID, it is crucial to evaluate both motor skills and physiological patterns.

If the patient exhibits physiological symptoms, it is essential to have the medical team involved. For example, gastrointestinal specialists rule out potential physiological causes (e.g., Eosinophilic Esophagitis (EOE), severe constipation, motility disorders, etc.). Once physiological causes are ruled out, it becomes imperative to address the identified issues and their presentation. Consider the below:

1. **Motor Skills:** Assessing the patient's ability to manipulate utensils, chew, and swallow effectively.
2. **Process Skills:** Evaluating the patient's planning, organizing, and sequencing abilities related to meal preparation and consumption.
3. **Social Interaction Skills:** Observing how the patient interacts with others during meal times, including communication and social behaviors.

Addressing these skills involves a comprehensive approach that may include therapeutic interventions to enhance motor coordination, strategies to improve meal preparation skills, and interventions to foster positive social interactions during meals. See more analysis of these sections in the treatment chapter.

Process Skills

Process skills involve the way an individual's thought and planning process is needed to perform an activity [14].

A patient's behavior will also be influenced by their process skills. Learning styles (tactile, visual, auditory) may influence how they take in information. Their ability to apply what they learn is often shaped by their own learning skills [15].

Timing Actions for ARFID patients can apply to planning meals by the patient or parent, which is an important process skill. Some patients can eat as long as food is presented at regular intervals, but if they (or their parents) need to do this independently, it often does not work. It is not uncommon for parents and patients to need explicit training and practice in how to time and plan their meals. Even college students, who for the first time have cafeteria passes, may find themselves missing meals due to overlapping classes, oversleeping, or struggling with overall time management [16].

Organizing Space and Objects for individuals with ARFID can be as basic as getting a lunch box or getting to the cafeteria lunch line in time. For college students, it may involve organizing a snack bag or meals. This aspect can be challenging, and patients may need specific training to build this skill. Often, college students with ARFID are taught to prep 10 snack bags (using paper sacks) over the weekend, writing down any perishable items they need to add on the front of the bag, and then get into the habit of grabbing the snack bag and placing it in their backpack before leaving their dorm or house. Teaching skills around organization is often an important development area for older teens and young adults [17]. Parents of patients with ARFID are often frustrated with the level of scaffolding their growing youth still requires in order to get enough nutrition, yet this support can be critically needed for their child or young adult to obtain the necessary life skills. Periods of transition are often some of the most important times to work with professionals to develop habits that will be health-sustaining.

Adapting Performance based on needs is crucial for ARFID patients. Often, when patients go home from the hospital on a behavior modification plan (e.g., Ladder Block Plan), they are advised to continue using it for 40–60 days at least through their first outpatient OT follow-up, and to also "pull it out" and use it again during times of transition. Many people will say that "things were going well until… I started school, started a job, got a girlfriend, etc." Changes in schedule and routines require adaptation, which can often be challenging for individuals who may not naturally prioritize food or be skillful in schedule management. Periods of transition are often some of the most important times to work with professionals to develop habits that will be health-supporting [18].

Social Interaction Skills can also impact feeding. If patients are uncomfortable eating at school or around certain noises, modifications may need to be made to ensure they eat successfully [19]. These modifications need to be examined on a case-by-case basis but may include things such as helping the client find a comfortable eating location (e.g., in a different spot within the school, with a white noise headset, etc.).

(v) **Client Factors (i.e., values, beliefs, spirituality, body functions, and body structures)**

There are many client and family factors that may impact their ability to eat. For example, if a patient has decided to become vegetarian to prevent animal cruelty, it may be difficult for them to eat meat. However, if meat is one of the family's staple foods, it may be clinically appropriate for them to resume eating it [20]. Further exploration and education often needs to take place, as many online images and messages about eating a certain way can be very intense. In some cases, the patient's media feeds and email subscriptions may need to be altered.

Certain festivals and traditions within a patient's religion may also affect their ability to consistently get enough nutrition [21]. In such cases, it is important to be culturally sensitive while providing education about what is physiologically required at that time. When medical recommendations conflict with religious customs, patients may need to seek further advice from their religious leaders. As medical professionals, it is important to state the medical need and document it. This information will be processed based on the individual's perceptions, values, and the recommendations of family members or other influential individuals.

There are times when a patient's true body functions impact their presentation [22]. For example, extensive constipation may influence both their fears (e.g., of a clean-out, of constipation) and their perceptions about eating (e.g., they may be afraid to eat certain foods that their doctor told them to avoid). For certain symptoms, some doctors may recommend an elimination diet or testing out gluten-free or dairy-free options. This change alone can sometimes cause enough weight loss to require hospitalization for malnutrition, bradycardia, or orthostasis. These patients often require education and relearning to address their nutritional deficits, and they may need to return to their typical way of eating to get enough nutrition.

Body structures can also impact issues related to nutrition. For instance, if someone has lost extensive weight and developed muscle atrophy, they may require specific interventions to regain strength and function. Patients with conditions like Ehlers-Danlos syndrome may have so many symptoms [23] that they limit their movement extensively and do not eat enough. Education about best recommendations for optimal physical function and the importance of salt intake becomes a priority in this case.

Occupational and Activity Analysis

Occupational and Activity Analysis is foundational in occupational therapy, guiding effective interventions across all patient populations. This process involves breaking down activities into their components to analyze steps and challenges, enabling the development of tailored treatment plans.

Occupational therapists evaluate the physical, cognitive, social, and environmental demands of activities to identify barriers to feeding and develop effective strategies [24]. For patients with ARFID, this analysis is particularly crucial. Eating and feeding are complex activities that involve multiple systems and skills. Understanding the intricacies of these tasks allows therapists to create interventions that are both effective and meaningful to the patient.

Components of Occupational and Activity Analysis for ARFID Patients

Task Analysis

Physical Demands: Assessing the capacity to sit with good posture, chew and swallow adequately, and the fine motor skills needed to manipulate food.

Cognitive Demands: Examining attention, memory, and problem-solving abilities essential for planning and completing meals.

Sensory Demands: Evaluating interactions with the appearance, texture, flavor, and smell of food, along with auditory or visual stimuli in the eating environment [25].

Social and Emotional Demands: Assessing the ability to eat in various social settings and understanding the emotional aspects of eating, including anxiety or discomfort in social contexts.

Environmental Analysis

Physical Environment: Examining the physical environment related to eating in both inpatient and outpatient settings. Identifying environments or times when eating is easier or more difficult provides valuable information for developing a treatment plan.

Social Environment: Assessing the level of family, caregiver, and social support available during meals. Determining the availability of primary caregivers for training and family meals, and the support required at home, school, or work.

Performance Analysis

Functional Abilities

Examining tone as it relates to posture and oral motor skills [26] is part of performance analysis. Assessing an individual's chewing and swallowing patterns while eating various food textures is an essential part of activity analysis. Even if an individual's tone is within normal limits, they may have developed postural or feeding mechanical habits (such as holding food in their mouth or delaying swallowing) that do not support optimal eating. Fine motor skills must also be examined, particularly in relation to the ability to access food (e.g., opening containers, cutting food) and feed themselves.

Prolonged inadequate nutrition can affect a patient's physical endurance [27] for sitting and feeding. Often, patients show improved capacity to eat when their posture is corrected. Attention and impulsivity during meal times can impact an individual's ability to sit through a meal. Those with memory deficits may require logs or methods for tracking their nutrition, as they might forget whether they have eaten. Some individuals can eat successfully when food is plated for them but struggle to plan their meals independently. They may require structured support and adaptive strategies to develop and maintain timely meal planning and eating habits. Additional training may be needed for some individuals to achieve consistent independence in obtaining adequate nutrition.

Individuals with ARFID, particularly those with the sensory subtype, may be sensitive to the taste, texture, smell, and appearance of food. They might also struggle with sensory aspects in their environment, such as sound or visual stimulation, especially in busy settings. Sometimes, a previously normal eater develops a pattern of becoming overwhelmed by large plates of food or by the contents of food. Examining the patient's sensory responses to their nutrition and environment can help build an appropriate step-by-step treatment plan.

Contextual Influences It is important to examine how the patient's environmental context (e.g., home, school, community) impacts their eating behaviors, including accessibility to preferred foods, mealtime routines, and distractions during meals [28]. Eating is often a social activity and holds significant cultural importance. In some cultures, parents may consider it a personal failure if their child is struggling with eating, and addressing their emotional processing is essential for the child's progress. It is crucial to examine how the patient interacts with and responds to family members during meals. Understanding these social dynamics, including interactions and conversations about food, provides valuable insights into the patient's eating behaviors and emotional responses. This analysis helps identify potential social and emotional barriers to optimal eating.

Adaptive Strategies Occupational therapists examine both the patient's perceived and observed barriers during meals and help develop strategies to address these challenges. A behavior modification plan may facilitate patient progress toward goals. Additionally, accommodations such as extra time to support meals, added structure during meals, and modifications in textures or drinks can help the patient meet full nutritional demands.

Support Needs Patients may require varying levels of support to ensure adequate nutrition, including supervision, prompting, or physical assistance [29]. The occupational therapist needs to consider the patient's self-management skills in maintaining consistent eating habits, including developing their ability to monitor and adjust their eating behaviors independently.

Occupational and activity analysis is an essential process in occupational therapy, providing the foundation for developing personalized and effective interventions for patients with ARFID. By thoroughly understanding the demands of eating and feeding tasks, therapists can create targeted strategies that address the unique challenges faced by these patients, ultimately supporting their progress and enhancing their participation in daily life.

Clinical and Professional Reasoning

Before examining the specifics of clinical and professional reasoning, it is valuable to understand how these concepts integrate with the practice domains and the overall approach of occupational therapy. Occupational therapists employ clinical and professional reasoning to tailor interventions effectively, ensuring that all aspects of a patient's condition and context are considered [30]. This reasoning process enables comprehensive and individualized care, which is essential when working with ARFID patients.

Professional reasoning in occupational therapy is the process used by practitioners to plan, direct, perform, and reflect on client care. This reasoning ensures that interventions are timely, relevant, and tailored to the patient's unique context, thereby influencing the effectiveness of the work carried out.

Clinical reasoning is defined as the process used by OT practitioners to understand the client's occupational needs, make decisions about intervention services, and think critically about what they do [31].

An occupational therapist uses both clinical and professional reasoning during the evaluation and throughout the treatment of the patient and their family.

When treating ARFID patients, an occupational therapist first needs to understand the ARFID subtype the patient has. See the psychology chapter for more details about this if the subtype is not provided. Knowing the correct subtype significantly influences which interventions are appropriate and the rationale for the interventions.

From a broader perspective, understanding how much time is available to work with a patient (inpatient or outpatient) assists in the development of the treatment plan and goal priorities. Professional reasoning involves using this information to plan and structure interventions effectively. For example, if a patient has significant medical instability, they may require a longer inpatient admission before they are ready for discharge. Similarly, outpatients may initiate services a couple of months prior to starting an out-of-state college or before a significant summer trip. Determining a timeline and goals, starting with the most critical or initial-step goals, is important. This process exemplifies professional reasoning by ensuring that interventions are timely, relevant, and tailored to the patient's unique context [32].

Addressing the patient's barriers to their optimal functioning is critical. One must look for both their stated barriers (e.g., early satiety, taking "too long" to eat) and those that are unstated (e.g., atypical oral motor issues). As later indicated, to optimize progress, stated barriers need to be addressed prior to the first feeding session. By having sessions where the patient is eating, the occupational therapist can address additional issues that occur during feeding and have the patient practice "in real time" the taught skills.

Understanding clinical and professional reasoning provides a solid foundation for the therapeutic process. Another critical component in delivering effective occupational therapy interventions is the therapeutic use of self. This involves the intentional application of a therapist's personal attributes and interpersonal skills to build rapport, motivate clients, and facilitate meaningful change. By integrating therapeutic use of self into practice, occupational therapists can enhance the efficacy of their interventions and support clients in achieving their goals.

Therapeutic Use of Self

In occupational therapy, "therapeutic use of self"is defined as the "planned use of his or her personality, insights, perceptions, and judgments as part of the therapeutic process" [33]. For an effective therapeutic use of self with patients who have ARFID, it is first important to establish a connection with the patient and family. Without rapport, any information shared will be less impactful. Therapeutic use of self is utilized to adapt the therapist's behaviors to what is needed for that patient. For example, an occupational therapist teaching oral motor skills may demonstrate how to eat something similar or how to use a NUK brush. If they have taught a skill such as relaxed posture with diaphragmatic breathing as a tool during meals, the therapist will model this behavior whenever supporting the client in feeding.

Therapeutic use of self supports the patient's progression by the therapist "playing the needed role" to facilitate the patient's progress. It supports a purposeful relationship between the therapist and the patient, promoting meaningful participation and progress in occupations that matter to the patient.

With ARFID patients, therapeutic use of self involves providing what the patient needs to progress. This may involve the role of educator, providing information about physiological recovery from malnutrition, techniques for overcoming barriers, and more. It may also involve the occupational therapist playing the role of a "relaxed, strong, and stable mealtime companion."

Therapeutic use of self may present in different forms over the course of treatment. Presenting as an individual who will "educate honestly about nutrition," talk to the patient truthfully (e.g., informing them if supplement quantities are changing), and provide ongoing calm and neutral support (without attachment to the results of any one meal) are often roles the OT takes on.

The following can add to the depth of therapeutic self and contribute to rapport building, facilitating learning and supporting patients in occupational therapy interventions. They can support the therapeutic process and environment.

Self-Care to Enhance Professional Effectiveness

As occupational therapists, it is your role to support patients in their healing process. The state of mind and well-being you bring into a patient's room can significantly impact the treatment session and the patient's progress. Reflecting on and understanding what enables you to maintain optimal physical, intellectual, and emotional energy is essential for effectively supporting your patients and yourself. Prioritizing self-care has an important impact on maintaining your well-being both professionally and personally and is a key component of actualizing therapeutic use of self [34].

Layer of Neutrality

An essential practice for clinicians and parents working with patients, including those with ARFID, is maintaining a layer of neutrality or dispassion. While "dispassion" might suggest emotional detachment, in this context, it refers to maintaining objectivity free from emotional biases. Educating parents of ARFID patients in this skill is crucial to supporting their child's progress. Parents can be coached to maintain a neutral demeanor, akin to a poker player concealing their hand, regarding their child's food-related progress.

Neutrality in emotional expression as it relates to food intake from the support team during meals is vital for patients with ARFID. Expressing overt excitement when the patient achieves milestones like eating more or trying new foods may inadvertently pressure them to perform consistently, which can be overwhelming. Conversely, displaying concern or dismay when the patient struggles can demotivate them. By remaining neutral throughout, treatment teams and parents help normalize eating behaviors as routine activities rather than extraordinary achievements. This helps the patient develop trust that the support will be with them regardless of how the meal goes. This is an important step for the patient's progress.

Neutral Language Use

In mental health, it has been established that non-judgmental communication facilitates greater patient progress compared to interactions perceived as judgmental [35]. As a clinician, the role involves accurately assessing and understanding the patient's situation to develop effective interventions. However, approaching interactions from a non-judgmental standpoint, particularly in educational contexts, often proves most therapeutic for patients.

Many patients, especially those in hospital settings, experience discomfort and recognize the need for change in their circumstances. As an occupational therapist, it is part of the role to help patients acknowledge their challenges without feeling judged, fostering a supportive environment conducive to growth. For instance, a patient may struggle with eating due to disrupted sleep patterns from excessive video gaming or substance use. Providing clinically informed education on the consequences of these behaviors, such as the impacts of sleep deprivation and substance use, without demonstrating moral judgments or biases can enhance openness to treatment.

Patients have often encountered similar information from family members, yet presenting it in a clinical, unbiased manner can facilitate better understanding and acceptance. Encouraging the development of new behavioral patterns both within and outside therapy sessions can empower patients to explore alternatives to their previous habits.

Unconditional Acceptance

To facilitate the development of any new behavior, it is crucial to begin with acceptance of the current situation. The therapist's ability to accept the patient "as they are" not only encourages honesty about their challenges but also establishes a foundation for skill-building. For many patients, acknowledging their current circumstances is necessary to making meaningful changes.

For instance, if a feeding plan prescribes three meals and two snacks per day but the patient consistently manages only two to four meals, accepting this reality is necessary. Once acceptance is established, the therapist can collaboratively explore strategies. These may involve adjusting the patient's sleep-wake cycle, scheduling meals around other activities (such as having lunch before a college math class), adapting to their established eating patterns by consolidating meals, and more. However, the initial and ongoing acceptance of the individual and their behaviors is essential before taking further therapeutic steps.

The theoretical foundation of occupational therapy provides essential insights into the physiological and emotional needs of patients with ARFID [36]. Understanding the impact of family dynamics and environmental factors on the patient, alongside comprehensive activity and task analysis, forms the cornerstone for effective evaluation and treatment planning.

Occupational Therapy Evaluation for ARFID Patients

Overview

Within the United States, depending on the state, Occupational Therapists (OTs) and Speech Therapists (STs) may treat feeding issues. In California, both OTs and STs can address Feeding Difficulties, with OTs requiring advanced practice certification for swallow assessment and interventions.

Evaluation Structure

Occupational Therapists aim to help patients reach their highest functional level by examining barriers to normal eating. For ARFID patients, these barriers may be physical (e.g., oral motor issues, early satiety, gagging, posture) or cognitive (e.g., fear of food, lack of food priority, not prioritizing nutrition). They can be impacted by family support, interactions, and environmental factors.

The structure for the first evaluation and treatment for ARFID patients includes:

- **Initial Evaluation**
- **Parent Meeting**
- **Meal Treatment Session** (typically preferred food parents have brought for outpatient or lunch for an inpatient). If inpatient this can be a separate follow-up treatment session
- **Follow-up Recommendations** (at least 5–20+ min after the meal to discuss the recommended initial feeding plan)

Initial Evaluation Components

- **Introduction to Occupational Therapy:** Explain OT's role in helping individuals reach their highest potential.
- **Patient and Parent Goals:** Understand both the patient's and parents' goals.
- **Oral Motor, Physical and Gross Motor Function Assessment:** Assess oral motor movement, and rule out tongue tie and structural anomalies. Evaluate the patient's baseline physical strength. Ensure gross motor skills and overall physical functioning are within normal limits by observing the patient walk across the room. Note any low tone, as this may impact oral motor skills.
- **Barrier Identification:** Identify barriers to normal eating as perceived by the patient and parents.

- **Introduction to Physiological Recovery Model:** Review the physiological impact of prolonged periods with insufficient nutrition and, at times, excessive activity. Explain the pathway of physiological recovery following inadequate nutrition, detailing the steps necessary to progress towards a state of thriving. A physiological recovery model description is in the Clinical Tools and Protocols Appendix A with a full size handout in Appendix N Chap. 22 Clinical Tools and Protocols.

Building rapport with the patient and family is an important component of the evaluation. This involves being present and patient, even if the patient is not speaking. It also includes observing verbal and non-verbal cues through active listening. Establishing trust is essential by showing that the therapist is supportive and reliable.

Key Questions

The first and last statements made by the occupational therapist are the most important during an evaluation or treatment session. After the obligatory name introduction, which may include "Nice to meet you", "patient" and "parent," you can say: "I'm [your name] from occupational therapy. Occupational therapy as a profession is committed to helping individuals reach their highest potential."

Looking at the patient directly and asking **"What is your goal of being here?"** is a powerful and relevant question. Many ARFID patients answer "to gain weight," "to learn to eat more," "to not have pain anymore," or if it is a patient with ARFID fear of aversive consequences, they may state their goal is "to not be afraid to eat." Then ask:

- "On a scale of 1-10, how much do you want to reach this goal?"
- "On a scale of 1-10, how much are you willing to work at it?"

If they want the goal more than they are willing to work at it, this is pointed out with a statement like, "Let's make a note that the desire is stronger than the willingness to work on it. This might be an issue; we will have to watch and see." The patient's desire to reach their goal and work towards it can be remembered by the clinician, and the patient may be reminded about it later when faced with challenges.

If the patient chooses a lower level (e.g., 5/10), you can skillfully ask: "What makes this so important to you that you did not choose a 4?" This can help validate that the patient does have some interest in getting better.

Addressing Barriers

- **Patient's Perspective:** Ask the patient about their perceived barriers to regular or adequate eating (e.g., fullness, fear of vomiting, nausea). You will then meet with the parents privately post the identification of the barriers to ensure that they will support what you will teach for overcoming the barriers, during the treatment session.
- **Parent Meeting:** Obtain a detailed history of the youth's eating patterns, early feeding difficulties, prior therapies, and recent changes. This is best done without the patient to avoid discouraging them. During this meeting, explain that parental attitude and support are key elements for the success of the treatment plan. Request that the parents support strategies taught and education provided by the OT and medical team when members are meeting with the patient and express any concerns privately to maintain a unified approach. Request them to respond neutrally to the patient's feeding presentation. This video (Video 6.1) provides a sample of how to explain neutrality to parents:

Video 6.1 Parent Guidance for Language Use https://youtu.be/0NrrwLhiN80

QR:

- Inform the parents that there will be regular individual meetings (often at the start of the treatment session), providing them an opportunity to fully express any concerns while also fully supporting the medical team.
- **Return to the Patient and Teach Initial Strategies**
- **Teach Strategies:** Introduce initial strategies to address barriers (these are fully described in the upcoming section).
- **Meal Plan:** Develop a plan for the first meal session, if outpatient give at least a 5 min break. Define the time of the meal and collect patient meal preferences if they are inpatient and there is time to request a specific food.
- **Encouragement:** Reassure the patient of the therapist's role in helping them improve their eating and overall well-being.

For an inpatient sample occupational therapy evaluation template, please refer to Appendix B in Chap. 22 Clinical Tools and Protocols.

References

1. Dahl-Popolizio S, Smith K, Day M, Muir S, Manard W. editors. Primary care occupational therapy: A quick reference guide. 2023. https://lane.stanford.edu/view/sul/14779812. https://link-springer-com.laneproxy.stanford.edu/book/10.1007/978-3-031-20882-9
2. Duncan EAS, editor. Skills for practice in occupational therapy. 2nd ed. Elsevier; 2023. https://lane.stanford.edu/view/bib/363671
3. Crepeau EB, Cohn ES, Schell BAB, editors. Willard & Spackman's occupational therapy. 11th ed. Wolters Kluwer Health/Lippincott Williams & Wilkins; 2009. https://lane.stanford.edu/view/bib/253012
4. Christiansen CH, Bass J, Baum CM. Occupational therapy: performance, participation, and Well-being. 4th ed. Routledge; 2014.
5. American Occupational Therapy Association. Occupational therapy scope of practice. Am J Occup Ther. 2021;75(Supplement_3):7513410020. https://doi.org/10.5014/ajot.2021.75S3005.
6. Mack RA, Stanton CE, Carney MR. The importance of including occupational therapists as part of the multidisciplinary team in the management of eating disorders: a narrative review incorporating lived experience. J Eat Disord. 2023;11(1):37. https://doi.org/10.1186/s40337-023-00763-6.
7. World Federation of Occupational Therapists. Statement on occupational therapy. WFOT; 2012. https://www.wfot.org/resources/statement-on-occupational-therapy
8. Gundersen C, Ziliak JP. Food insecurity and health outcomes. Health Aff. 2015;34(11):1830–9. https://doi.org/10.1377/hlthaff.2015.0645.
9. Borsarini B, Pappaianni E, Micali N. Locked down with my eating disorder: A retrospective study on the impact of COVID-19 lockdown on adolescents with eating disorders. J Eat Disord. 2023;11:71. https://doi.org/10.1186/s40337-023-00792-1.
10. Xiong J, Lipsitz O, Nasri F, Lui LMW, Gill H, Phan L, Chen-Li D, Iacobucci M, Ho R, Majeed A, McIntyre RS. Impact of COVID-19 pandemic on mental health in the general population: A systematic review. J Affect Disord. 2020;277:55–64. https://doi.org/10.1016/j.jad.2020.08.001. Epub 2020 Aug 8. PMID: 32799105; PMCID: PMC7413844
11. Keski-Rahkonen A, Ruusunen A. Avoidant-restrictive food intake disorder and autism: epidemiology, etiology, complications, treatment, and outcome. Curr Opin Psychiatry. 2023;36(6):438–42. https://doi.org/10.1097/YCO.0000000000000896.
12. Shove E, Trentmann F, Wilk R, editors. Time, consumption and everyday life: practice, materiality and culture. 1st ed. Routledge; 2009. https://doi.org/10.4324/9781003087236.
13. Duncan EAS, editor. Foundations for practice in occupational therapy. 6th ed. Elsevier; 2020.
14. American Occupational Therapy Association. Occupational therapy practice framework: domain and process (4th). Am J Occup Ther. 2020;74(Suppl. 2):7412410010. https://doi.org/10.5014/ajot.2020.74S2001.
15. Bhagat A, Vyas R, Singh T. Students awareness of learning styles and their perceptions to a mixed method approach for learning. Int J Appl Basic Med Res. 2015;5(Suppl 1):S58–65. https://doi.org/10.4103/2229-516X.162281.
16. Wongprawmas R, Sogari G, Menozzi D, Mora C. Strategies to promote healthy eating among university students: A qualitative study using the nominal group technique. Front Nutr. 2022;9:821016. https://doi.org/10.3389/fnut.2022.821016.
17. Freedman S. Developing college skills in students with autism and Asperger's syndrome. Jessica Kingsley Publishers; 2010. https://doi.org/10.5040/9781849058462.
18. Hall KK, Shoemaker-Hunt S, Hoffman L, Earl T, Katapodis N, Schneiderman S. Making healthcare safer III: A critical analysis of existing and emerging patient safety practices [Internet]. Agency for Healthcare Research and Quality (US); 2020. https://www.ncbi.nlm.nih.gov/books/NBK555526/.

19. Kluckow H, Telfer J, Abraham S. Should we screen for misophonia in patients with eating disorders? A report of three cases. Int J Eat Disord. 2014;47(5):558–61. https://doi-org.laneproxy.stanford.edu/10.1002/eat.22245
20. Bardone-Cone AM, Fitzsimmons-Craft EE, Harney MB, Maldonado CR, Lawson MA, Smith R, Robinson DP. The inter-relationships between vegetarianism and eating disorders among females. J Acad Nutr Diet. 2012;112(8):1247–52. https://doi.org/10.1016/j.jand.2012.05.007.
21. Akgül S, Derman O, Kanbur NÖ. Fasting during Ramadan: a religious factor as a possible trigger or exacerbator for eating disorders in adolescents. Int J Eat Disord. 2014;47(8):905–10. https://doi-org.laneproxy.stanford.edu/10.1002/eat.22255
22. Rosh JR, Heitlinger LA, Rosenfeld WD, editors. Clinical GI challenges in the adolescent, vol. 27, No. 1. American Academy of Pediatrics; 2016. https://lane.stanford.edu/view/sul/13048969
23. Lee M, Strand M. Ehlers-Danlos syndrome in a young woman with anorexia nervosa and complex somatic symptoms. Int J Eat Disord. 2018;51(3):281–4. https://doi-org.laneproxy.stanford.edu/10.1002/eat.22815
24. Case-Smith J, Allen AS, Pratt PN, editors. Occupational therapy for children. 3rd ed. Mosby; 1996. https://lane.stanford.edu/view/bib/88327
25. Nimbley E, Golds L, Sharpe H, Gillespie-Smith K, Duffy F. Sensory processing and eating behaviours in autism: A systematic review. European Eating Disorders Review: J Eating Disorders Association. 2022;30(5):538–59. https://doi.org/10.1002/erv.2920.
26. Harris SR. Congenital hypotonia: clinical and developmental assessment. Developmental Medicine & Child Neurology. 2008;50(11):889–92. https://doi.org/10.1111/j.1469-8749.2008.03097.x.
27. Smith L, López Sánchez GF, Fernandez-Egea E, Ford T, Parris C, Underwood BR, Butler L, Barnett Y, Trott M, Koyanagi A. Eating disorders and physical multimorbidity in the English general population. Eat Weight Disord. 2023;28(1):72. https://doi-org.laneproxy.stanford.edu/10.1007/s40519-023-01600-0
28. Lukas L, Buhl C, Schulte-Körne G, Sfärlea A. Family, friends, and feelings: the role of relationships to parents and peers and alexithymia in adolescents with anorexia nervosa. J Eat Disord. 2022;10(1):143. https://doi-org.laneproxy.stanford.edu/10.1186/s40337-022-00661-3
29. Kim YK, Di Martino JM, Nicholas J, Rivera-Cancel A, Wildes JE, Marcus MD, Sapiro G, Zucker N. Parent strategies for expanding food variety: reflections of 19,239 adults with symptoms of avoidant/restrictive food intake disorder. Int J Eat Disord. 2022;55(1):108–19. https://doi.org/10.1002/eat.23639.
30. Shafaroodi N, Kamali M, Parvizy S, Mehraban AH, O'Toole G. Factors affecting clinical reasoning of occupational therapists: a qualitative study. Med J Islam Repub Iran. 2014;28:8. https://lane.stanford.edu/view/pubmed/25250253
31. Mattingly C. What is clinical reasoning? Am J Occup Ther. 1991;45(11):979–86. https://doi.org/10.5014/ajot.45.11.979.
32. Summers BE, Laver KE, Nicks RJ, Andrew NE, Barr CJ, Jolliffe L, Lannin NA. Patient functional independence and occupational therapist time-use in inpatient services: patient demographic and clinical correlates. Hong Kong J Occupation Therapy: HKJOT. 2021;34(2):73–82. https://doi.org/10.1177/15691861211018758.
33. Taylor RR, Lee SW, Kielhofner G, Ketkar M. Therapeutic use of self: a nationwide survey of practitioners' attitudes and experiences. Am J Occup Ther. 2009;63(2):198–207. https://doi-org.laneproxy.stanford.edu/10.5014/ajot.63.2.198.
34. Posluns K, Gall TL. Dear mental health practitioners, take care of yourselves: a literature review on self-care. Int J Adv Couns. 2020;42(1):1–20. https://doi.org/10.1007/s10447-019-09382-w.
35. Dews SA, Daley R, Bansal A, Preston J, Bohm N. The power of language: how to bridge the gap between healthcare research and patients—A scoping review. Curr Med Res Opin. 2024;40(2):279–91. https://doi.org/10.1080/03007995.2023.2295984.
36. Willman R, Hobbs M, Thomas JJ. The potential role of occupational therapy in the treatment of avoidant/restrictive food intake disorder. Int J Eat Disord. 2024;57:1985–90. https://doi.org/10.1002/eat.24199. Advance online publication.

Chapter 7
Occupational Therapy Strategies to Overcome Barriers to Full Nutrition

Strategies to Overcome Barriers to Full Nutrition

Section 1: Addressing Stated Barriers

Introduction

Just as firefighters train extensively before facing a fire, addressing known barriers to eating in patients requires thorough preparation and proactive strategies. Reported barriers that impact feeding should be addressed prior to the first meal. Additional barriers that arise during or around meals should be addressed as they are observed, ideally in between mealtime treatment sessions. Though this section has been written by an occupational therapist and therefore inherently has an occupational therapy lens, it is recognized that many medical treatment team members may find these strategies useful to teach while working with patients.

General Issues

This includes issues that may arise for all ARFID subtypes.

Nausea
Early Satiety or Stomach Pain

While most of the research in managing nausea has been in post-surgical, cancer and pregnancy patients [1, 2] many of the same techniques can help individuals with ARFID for addressing nausea management.

Nausea can present a significant barrier to normal eating, and understanding its various causes is helpful for effective management. It is important to assess the patterns of nausea by asking questions such as, "When does the nausea typically occur?

A. B. Sinha et al., *Comprehensive Clinical Care for Adolescents with Avoidant/Restrictive Food Intake Disorder (ARFID)*,
https://doi.org/10.1007/978-3-031-92232-9_7

How long does it last?" Patients should be introduced to the three primary causes of nausea that impacts feeding and asked to identify which type(s) they experience.

Primary Types of Nausea That Impact Feeding

1. **Morning Nausea:**
   - Occurs due to inadequate nutrition from previous days, similar to morning sickness in pregnancy.
   - Resolves with consistent nutrition over weeks to months.

> Emphasize nighttime snacks and regular morning meals.

2. **Nausea while Eating or After:**
   - Often linked to discomfort with fullness or constipation.
   - Typically resolves within 3–10 days after reaching nutritional goals.

> Monitor for constipation and adjust meal sizes gradually.

3. **Nausea Related to Anxiety or Emotions:**
   - Common in patients with anxiety disorders.
   - Coexists with physiological nausea but requires distinct management.
   - Inquire if nausea occurs in moments of stress (e.g., tests) or sometimes upon seeing food

> Teach relaxation techniques like abdominal breathing and straw breath to manage anxiety-related nausea.

Collecting Background Information on Nausea:

Vestibular Nausea: Though this nausea type does not impact eating (except as it may lead to food avoidance around car rides), collecting this information helps in understanding if the patient has a baseline tendency towards nausea which may mean that the individual needs ongoing nausea strategies

- Triggered by motion or positional changes.
- Indicates sensitivity to vestibular stimuli.

Techniques for Nausea:

- **Breathing Techniques for nausea related to anxiety (with or without nausea)** [2]:
- **Abdominal Breathing with loose body posture** (Video 7.1)**:**

Video 7.1 Abdominal Breathing with Loose Body Posture

https://youtu.be/j9n46sLm3Yc

QR:

- **Straw Breath:** Straw breath (Video 7.2) emphasizes a slower exhalation. It includes a breath in through the nose and a breath out slowly through pursed lips

Video 7.2 Straw Breath

3 https://youtu.be/QYgCv977-K8

QR:

Does Breath Pattern Impact Anxiety Level?
Physiologically, the heart rate increases during inhalation and decreases during exhalation. In healthy individuals at baseline the heart rate variability includes longer exhalations. Research supports that longer exhalations can promote vagal tone and relaxation [3].

Other Techniques:

- **Body Positions:** Advise sitting upright during meals to reduce nausea; ensure relaxation of feet, knees, shoulders, and jaw.
- **Environmental Factors:** Control room temperature and avoid overheating, clothing layers may need to be removed.
- **Acupressure Point (Nei Guan—P6)** [4] (Fig. 7.1):
  - Locate three finger breadths below the wrist on the inner forearm.
  - Apply firm pressure to relieve nausea and motion sickness.
  - Instruction: Demonstrate proper technique and provide visual aids if available.
  - **Consideration:** Sometimes the tendons are fibrous or connected. In such cases, scoop under the tendon on the ulnar side to access this point effectively.
  - For a visual demonstration of how to locate and apply pressure to the P6 acupressure point, please refer to the accompanying digital media (Video 7.3).

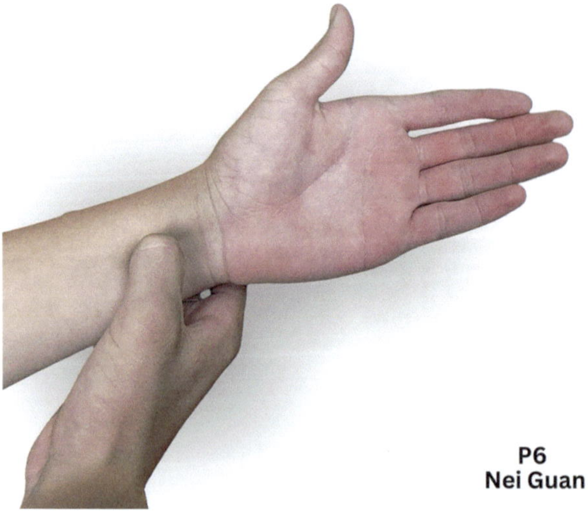

Fig. 7.1 Acupressure Point (Nei Guan—P6) for addressing nausea

Video 7.3 Pressure Point P6 for Nausea
https://youtu.be/QEab3aqWf40

QR:

Additional Tools and Remedies:

- **Acu-bands** [5]: Use the principle of acupressure with bands. May not be as effective for individuals without a gap between their middle two tendons.
- **Relief Band** [6]: A therapeutic device approved for reducing nausea and vomiting. It uses pulses to stimulate the median nerve and rebalance nerve messages to alleviate symptoms. Our institution lends these out for trial use and they are sold in the hospital gift shop.
- **Aromatherapy** [7]: Use of essential oils such as mint or lavender. Smelling coffee grounds can be used to help patient shift their smell sense when scent feels overwhelming
- **Alcohol Pads** [8]: Inhaling isopropyl alcohol helps alleviate nausea for some patients.
- **Ginger Chews and Teas** [9, 10]: Ginger chews, ginger ale, and mint or ginger tea can help with nausea for some patients.

For an explanation of these strategies on addressing nausea, please refer to the accompanying digital media (Video 7.4).

Video 7.4 Summary of Additional Techniques for Nausea
https://youtu.be/bF1UQ42F78U

QR:

By addressing nausea proactively with targeted strategies, occupational therapists can enhance the eating experience and overall well-being of ARFID patients.

Addressing Early Satiety or Stomach Pain

Any ARFID patient could report getting full easily or stomach upset as a barrier to normal eating. For patients with early satiety or stomach discomfort, learning a pressure point for stomach fullness and using hot packs post-meals can be very helpful. It is also important to rule out constipation which can be a side-effect of malnutrition. If constipation is present, alert the medical team and address it as an occupational therapist (see Chap. 22 Clinical Tools and Protocols Appendix D, E, F page). Some patients may not report this as an initial barrier, but it may emerge as meal plans increase.

- **Hot Packs** Hot packs or heating pads are a useful tool for individuals feeling stomach discomfort [11] which could be perceived as fullness or pain. They are usually the most effective post-meals as during the meal they sometimes distract from the eating process.
- **Pressure Point for Early Satiety or Fullness** The pressure point called the "Hand Valley Point"LI-4 [12, 13] (Fig. 7.2) (Video 7.5) is located about three of the patient's thumb tips into the muscle belly, as pictured. Practitioners should learn to find it on themselves and others and then teach patients. This pressure point is useful when the patient feels early satiety, discomfort, or fullness. Have them practice as they would during a meal, pressing it themselves for 1 min with 5 pounds of pressure and letting their breath move in and out. If they are using it during a meal, they should then take more bites (if still eating). If they do not feel relief, have them use the other hand as well and double-check their pressure level to make sure it is not too light to be effective.

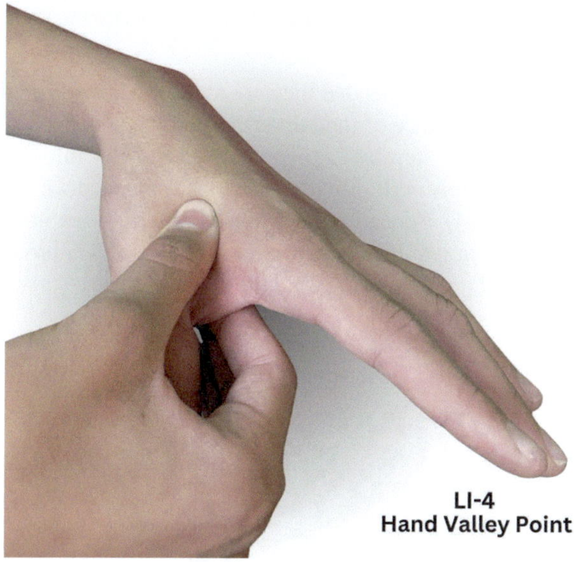

Fig. 7.2 Acupressure point (Hand Valley Point LI-4) for addressing early satiety or fullness

Video 7.5 LI-4 Pressure Point for Early Satiety or Fullness

https://youtu.be/fboYJdbB4HA

QR:

Issues Related to ARFID Subtypes

Though the barriers for the Sensory Eaters and Low Interest Eaters may become more revealed when observing a feeding session, providing a framework for how to approach feeding can help these patients in a needed shift in attitude towards eating more diversely or eating enough. The below education is recommended prior to the first meal during the evaluation:

ARFID- Sensory Eaters or Picky Eaters

If a patient mentions that they are a picky eater during the evaluation, educate them on the importance of food diversity and the concept of food jags, and reassure them that there are step-by-step approaches to help. Inform the patient that the occupational therapist will provide additional guidance when the opportunity arises to eat together [14]. Education for picky eaters will be explored further in the next section.

For a sample of this education, this Video 7.6 provides information that can be presented at the time of evaluation.

Video 7.6 Food Rotation to Avoid Food Jags

https://youtu.be/W7Eui4hpKrY

QR:

ARFID- Low Interest

Individuals with ARFID—low interest tend to not get enough nutrition to sustain themselves and may have dulled bodily cues related to eating. After reviewing the physiological recovery model during the evaluation, discuss their eating philosophy. This discussion is important, but particularly when their eating philosophy differs from their parents, the realization of the impact of their food views and the way they live is especially important for the patient and parent to realize.

A discussion with the patient about whether they "live to eat" or "eat to live" at the time of evaluation can help the patient understand that they may see nutrition primarily as a source of sustenance, rather than enjoyment or comfort. This perspective means they might not seek out food as often as is beneficial to their body. Understanding how they view food can guide treatment and educate caregivers, helping the patient recognize the need to schedule meals into their day just like school, work, and homework.

Parents of these teens are often frustrated that "they still need help," but part of the required assistance to the youth may involve training them to make food a priority. Challenge the patient to observe how regular eating impacts their body energetically.

For more information, refer to the educational Video 7.7 on this topic.

Video 7.7 Regular Meal Schedule

https://youtu.be/ArIbaUqysbk

QR:

ARFID- Fear of Aversive Consequences

Patients with ARFID who fear aversive consequences may experience a range of challenges. Addressing these issues before the first feeding session is critical to ensuring compliance and facilitating progress.

Addressing Fear of Emesis

Patients with emetophobia have a fear of eating due to the belief that it will lead to vomiting [15]. This fear may stem from a past experience with vomiting, witnessing someone else vomit, or even just the anticipation of it. Interestingly, most individuals with this fear rarely, if ever, actually vomit, yet the fear remains strong [16]. They may worry that eating too much will cause emesis, even if it has never happened before.

It's important to identify if patients have this fear, as it can be effectively addressed with the right training. A fear of vomiting is one of the most common concerns among those with a fear of aversive consequences. Additionally, this fear might not initially be present in patients with ARFID, particularly those with low interest or sensory-related issues, but it can develop as they begin to expand their diet. Addressing this fear once acknowledged can prevent it from becoming a more entrenched worry. For these patients, techniques to manage this fear might not be introduced initially but may become relevant as their meal plan progresses.

Research has been done about the impact on abdominal breathing to decrease rumination and it has been found to be an effective treatment when taught correctly [17, 18]. It also addresses vomiting (and does prevent vomiting in rumination patients) but has not been researched outside of the context of rumination. The same mechanisms that allow patients to avoid rumination through diaphragmatic breathing, also work for avoiding emesis. Physiologically, one can only have emesis if the breath pattern is superficial. Often when this gets coupled with bent or rigid posture it is easier for it to happen physiologically. One cannot throw up if their body is loose and if their breath is diaphragmatic.

In order to teach the patient, ask, "Would you like to learn the secret to not vomiting?" First, move the patient to a chair. Check the patient's baseline breathing pattern and evaluate whether it is superficial or diaphragmatic by having them take a breath in and out. If their breath pattern is superficial (as is the case for many individuals), it doesn't necessarily mean that the patient *will* vomit. However, if they are very nauseous and breathing superficially, physiologically it is possible to vomit. If they are able to relax their posture and breath abdominally, it won't be possible to vomit.

Digital Video: How to Avoid Vomiting

View this Video 7.8 to see how this can be explained to a patient.

Video 7.8 Abdominal Breathing with Loose Body Posture to Prevent Vomiting and Address Fear of Vomiting

https://youtu.be/tgzIOto80u0

QR:

Show the patient the two below positions (i.e., leaning forward (Fig. 7.3) and sitting upright (Fig. 7.4)) and ask them to guess in which position the person is more likely to throw up (usually this can be done not through a picture but through the position of the therapist's body position/demonstration). The answer to this is that person A, who has their shoulders elevated, their body tight, and a forward posture, is more likely to throw up.

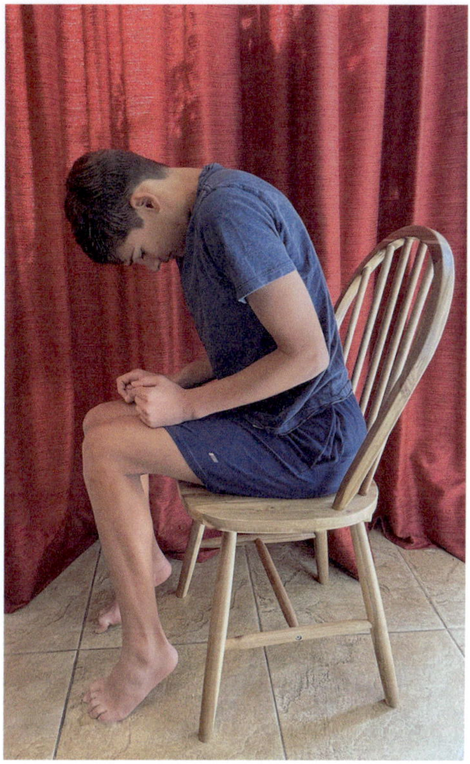

Fig. 7.3 Individual sitting in hunched position

Posturally, to Avoid Emesis, Keep the Body Loose Check in for body tension at four points: head (keep jaw loose), shoulders (keep relaxed, down, and relaxed, you may want to place a pillow behind the back), knees (knees should be so relaxed that if they were bumped they would move), and toes (relaxed and on the floor). If toes cannot touch the floor, place a small stool that feet can be rested on. Not only will this reduce the feeling of nausea, but it also tends to help individuals focus better, which is useful for eating. If it is hard to sit with good posture or is less comfortable, place a pillow behind the back (Fig. 7.5). Most individuals who tend to slouch at baseline do better with a pillow behind their back.

If the patient learns abdominal breathing easily, encourage them to start practicing abdominal breathing and loose body posture for 5–10 breaths prior to eating and two other times during the day and before bed.

If it is difficult for them to learn in a seated position, have them practice abdominal breathing while lying down. Have the patient place a pen or a small stuffed animal near their belly button. Encourage them to lift the item up as they breathe in and lower it as they breathe out. Encourage the patient to practice to start to build confidence (if hospitalized, they can practice it when vitals are taken). Building this skill often takes a couple days of practice. Once the patient can utilize abdominal breathing consistently while lying, have them practice in a seated position per above

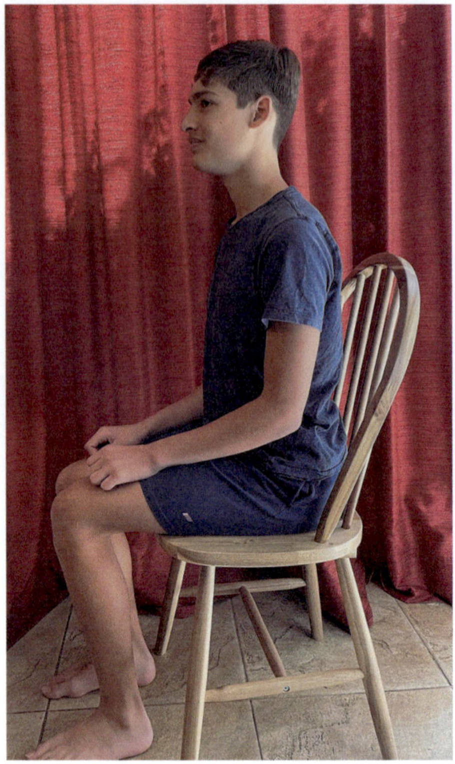

Fig. 7.4 Individual sitting in relaxed upright position

instructions. Review abdominal breathing at all non-meal sessions and during the meals as needed. The goal is to become confident in the use of this technique in-between meals so that if they "have a moment of need" where they need the strategy to prevent vomiting, they can "pull it out and use it" effectively.

What is Superficial Breathing? What is Abdominal Breathing?
Superficial breathing involves the chest rising with inhalation and falling with exhalation, which contrasts with abdominal breathing where the abdomen expands during inhalation and contracts during exhalation.
Why Deep Breathing and Abdominal Breathing Are Not the Same Thing
Deep breathing can still be superficial; it's possible to take deep breaths that primarily move the chest rather than the abdomen. Superficial deep breaths are less effective on a physiological level and do not prevent vomiting. In contrast, diaphragmatic (or abdominal) breathing offers additional health benefits, such as superior modulation of cardiac autonomic function. This enhances the heart's ability to adapt to physiological demands, offering greater benefits to patients compared to generalized deep breathing techniques [19].

Vomiting

If a patient is having regular emesis, medical causes (e.g., cannabinoid hyperemesis syndrome, hyperemesis syndrome, cancer, cyclic vomiting syndrome) must be ruled out prior to occupational therapy beginning treatment.

Sometimes it is primarily a morning vomiting scenario that improves as the patient is able to take in nutrition throughout the day. At other times, an individual with ARFID could have developed a physiological pattern of vomiting anytime they eat.

If someone is vomiting two or more times per day, it is useful to separate fluids and viscous foods (e.g., yogurt, fruit cups) from solid foods. It is useful to have someone sit with them while they work on developing the skill of not vomiting. Depending on the patient's baseline, the goal is to either initially extend time without vomiting or to decrease the frequency of vomiting. The occupational therapist will sit with the patient during the meal and for at least 20 min after the meal. If the vomiting is very frequent, sometimes a behavior modification plan is created to reinforce going longer periods without vomiting.

Strategies to Prevent Vomiting Watch the Video 7.9 for a step-by-step guide on physiological strategies to prevent vomiting.

Video 7.9 Abdominal Breathing with Loose Body Posture to Prevent Vomiting

https://youtu.be/eHa0u3QmBIU

Any patterns that relate to vomiting (e.g., running to the bathroom, vomiting in a bag or garbage) must be eliminated with absolute reassurance that any messes will be cleaned up. Breathing abdominally does not decrease nausea (unless the nausea is anxiety-related), and frequently the nausea strategies are quite helpful in addition to the strategies to avoid emesis. As patients practice, they will initially go longer without emesis, and their frequency of emesis will decrease until it is completely eliminated.

A Word about Buckets, Trash Cans and Toilets

In a hospital setting, if someone mentions they are going to throw up, a pink bucket or an emesis bag is typically delivered promptly. Within the home setting it is a garbage can or a run to the bathroom. Unfortunately, this can create a negative association with these items. It may become a pattern for patients to anticipate vomiting, feel nauseous, or spit into these receptacles. To break this association and reduce vomiting behaviors, it's essential not to provide patients with objects associated with emesis or spitting. Instead, reassure them that any vomiting incidents will be cleaned up promptly and without complaint. This initial adjustment may be challenging for patients, but it's crucial to support them step-by-step in breaking this habit and association.

Fear of Reflux

Gastroesophageal reflux (GER) or gastroesophageal reflux disease (GERD) in children can cause symptoms such as heartburn, regurgitation, and nausea or vomiting, often occurring after meals. Medical causes for reflux should be ruled out. Youth often become scared that it will happen again after the first incident. The medical team often rules out and addresses constipation. Learning to breathe abdominally as their dominant breath pattern helps to reduce reflux [20], and practicing abdominal breathing with a loose body posture after it occurs helps prevent it from happening again.

Fear of Rumination

Rumination syndrome involves the repeated regurgitation of undigested or partially digested food from the stomach, followed by re-chewing and swallowing or spitting out the food. This occurs involuntarily, without effort or intention. The regurgitated food tastes similar to regular food and is not acidic like vomit.

Similar strategies to those used to prevent vomiting can effectively manage rumination: maintaining a loose body posture and practicing abdominal breathing [21]. If the patient reports or describes rumination as a concern at the time of evaluation, it is important to teach this strategy prior to an eating session and to tell them that there is a treatment for food repeatedly coming up. A diagnosis for rumination is symptom and medical history based and can be made by the medical and psychiatry teams. Further information about treating rumination can be found in Cllinical Tools and Protocols Appendix C.

Fear of Constipation

At times, ARFID patients may present with additional gastrointestinal concerns which can significantly impact their eating behaviors [22, 23]. A patient who has undergone a gastrointestinal clean-out may develop a fear of eating, worried that eating will necessitate another clean-out or lead to further constipation. At other times, constipation becomes an issue over the course of treatment [24]. When constipation is a fear, an introduction about addressing constipation and the importance of eating regularly to support motility needs to occur at the time of the evaluation with assurances that more education will be provided.

Educating patients about the main components of bowel health, keeping stool soft enough to push, toilet sitting at the right time, and having proper coordination [25], can alleviate some of their fears. It's also important that they can assess the bathroom at any time. Introducing tools like the Bristol Stool Chart [26] for communication with physicians and a footstool [27] for better toileting posture can be helpful. For more detailed information and additional training and handouts on these topics, please refer to Chap. 22 Clinical Tools and Protocols Appendix D, E and F.

Fear of Choking

Some individuals with ARFID may report pseudodysphagia, a fear of choking [28], often arising after a choking incident or witnessing someone else choke. This fear can lead them to restrict their diet to soft foods and liquids, potentially resulting in weight loss requiring medical intervention. They may constantly worry about choking during meals.

As with all patients, medical causes for choking must first be ruled out [29, 30] by the medical team. Procedures like endoscopy, videofluroscopic swallow study (VFSS) or fiberoptic endoscopic evaluation of swallowing (FEES) may be necessary to confirm normal swallowing function and reassure the patient.

Before the first feeding session, it's crucial to address what to do in case of choking (Video 7.10). Teach the patient that if they can speak clearly, they are not choking. Giving them something concrete to say like "A,B,C" or "1,2,3" helps when used during meals if explained in advance. Teach them (and practice this only once at the evaluation) to lift their hands above their head and cough loudly if they cannot speak. Additionally, teach them the universal choking sign and how to dial 911.

Video 7.10 Strategies for Fear of Choking

https://youtu.be/uxnEkbE4ZeU

Fear of Pain

Some individuals become fearful of eating due to ongoing pain issues, GI symptoms, or fears of allergies. These issues must start to be addressed prior to the first feeding session with additional training throughout.

When an individual has stomach pain impacting their eating, a full gastrointestinal work-up is critical to rule out any physical causes prior to occupational therapy sessions. Sometimes, the individual gets diagnosed with functional abdominal pain or a pain syndrome that is not going to quickly change [31]. In these cases, addressing the nature of the pain and providing education about malnutrition is important. Use of the “Hand Valley Point” and hot packs can be reviewed.

If the patient has chronic pain, it is essential to have a private discussion with the parents or guardians to engage them in the treatment plan and help with buy-in. Engaging the family early is crucial, as parents may feel frustrated, protective, or defensive. Gaining their support for occupational therapy (OT) intervention is key [32] and should begin before the first meal. At that point there should then be a conversation with the caregivers and patient that acknowledges the patient’s experience with pain and prepares them for understanding the nature of chronic pain.

Chronic pain is pain that lasts longer than the normal healing period, typically extending beyond 3 to 6 months. It can fluctuate, ranging from mild to severe [33]. Unlike acute pain, chronic pain has a longer trajectory, and when it leads to a significant reduction or change in diet, it becomes incongruent with maintaining health. When educating the family, emphasize that regardless of the pain’s cause, addressing nutrition is essential if it significantly impacts the patient’s health. While the ongoing pain can be frustrating, parents typically appreciate the support and education on improving their child’s nutrition.

Research indicates that those who are happiest while experiencing chronic pain do two things: they do not give up hope for a cure, and they live life fully anyway [34]. (see Chap. 22 Clinical Tools and Protocols Appendix M for full size hand-out). Teach that not giving up hope for a cure, when GI has ruled out immediate causes, often means trying one item at a time to see if it impacts chronic pain (e.g., a different regime to address constipation/bowel health, different medication, a different therapy like acupuncture or chiropractic care). Educate them about the importance of finding a way to get adequate nutrition despite the pain which can be addressed a step at a time while still acknowledging and working to address the pain. At times, developing a customized pain log can help patients increase their functional activity (see Appendix G).

Fear of Food Variety and Food Avoidance Due to Recommended Special Diets

Patients with stomach pain or other medical issues may have tried various special diets (e.g., elimination, gluten-free, dairy-free) in an effort to manage their symptoms. However, these diets may not work [35] and can sometimes lead to malnutrition because eliminating foods can result in too few options or the consumption of less calorically dense foods. This can create a caloric deficit, further exacerbating the patient's nutritional status [36].

Aligning with the medical team and then reassuring patients that they have a history of eating diverse foods and that their body is capable of digesting previously consumed foods is important. This can help alleviate some of the stress and anxiety surrounding food and pain. It's crucial to acknowledge that the perception that certain foods exacerbate pain has been built up over time.

When ARFID patients receive medical "permission" to reintroduce previously eliminated foods, many are eager to do so. This reintroduction can often be both a stressor and a relief. The stress comes from the ingrained belief that certain foods may trigger pain, while the relief comes from the possibility of diversifying their diet and enjoying foods they have avoided for a while.

Fear of Foods Due to Perceived Allergies or Sensitivities

Some patients experience decreased nutrition and reduced eating ability due to a reaction to an allergen or fear of potential allergens [37]. Before the occupational therapist works with these patients they must have clear information from the medical team regarding the status of their true allergies. This information must then be presented at the evaluation prior to the first feeding session with the reassurance that the occupational therapist will work with them to gradually expand food variety within the realm of medical recommendations. Again, talking to the parents privately prior to this education is critical for it to be effective.

> Addressing a patient's perceived and known obstacles prior to feeding sessions while providing relevant tools and insights helps acknowledge what the patient has experienced while providing solution-based strategies. Once this step is complete, the occupational therapist will then examine the unstated obstacles to eating during feeding sessions.

Section 2: Exploring Additional Barriers Through Postural and Oral Motor Analysis

A thorough analysis of postural and oral motor patterns is crucial for a comprehensive treatment plan [38]. Identifying and addressing subtle aspects of a patient's eating process, such as posture and chewing patterns, allows occupational therapists to uncover additional barriers and develop a more effective treatment plan.

> A clinician's scope of practice can vary by region. If examining physiology or oral motor skills, it is important to determine whether it is in the scope of practice of your professional realm. Dysphagia is rare among adolescent ARFID patients, and the scope of this section does not include detailed evaluations for dysphagia. If concerns arise, request a bedside swallow evaluation and consider additional instrumental testing (e.g., videofluoroscopy, endoscopy) if needed. Be sure to do a warm handoff with the team members conducting testing and ask them to provide reassurance about normal swallow function if the tests are within normal limits.

Eating with the Patient

The most important action an occupational therapist can take to progress feeding is to be present while the patient is eating, actively observing their posture, oral motor mechanics, behavioral patterns, and parent interactions [39]. Where possible, it can be therapeutic for the therapist to have some food at the same time, this allows the therapist to demonstrate chewing patterns and creates a more natural atmosphere for the patient than simply observing them eating.

The occupational therapist's role is to create a comfortable and supportive environment. While the patient is eating, it is important to keep the conversation on neutral, light, and pleasant topics. Suitable topics include travel, places they would like to visit, their pets (as long as their pets are healthy and haven't recently passed away), movies, video games, and music. Avoid topics related to politics, their family, or school, as these can be sources of stress.

Before the first eating experience, advise the parents to follow this same routine. During the evaluation, the occupational therapist will have already discussed with the parents the importance of maintaining a "layer of neutrality." Frequently, parents will require additional training and debriefing on how to maintain a light atmosphere during meals. It can also be helpful to instruct the parents not to comment on the quantity or quality of the food, but to remain supportive.

If the patient normally watches movies or videos while eating and the parent is comfortable with this, it is acceptable to continue this practice if it doesn't negatively impact their feeding quantity or abilities. Sometimes a meal with and without media will be needed to determine this. When using a screen, ensure that it is kept at or above eye level, using a stand or other method to elevate, if necessary. This supports good posture. For some patients, playing tabletop games during the meal can also work if it doesn't cause delays in taking bites. Sometimes family members can strategically delay the next game play until a bite is taken.

If the occupational therapist has already taught the strategies that will help the patient, reinforce them as needed during the meal. If a new issue arises, provide minor teaching during the meal and follow up with the patient between eating sessions. Whenever possible, debrief with the patient with a 5–20 min gap after the meal was completed to discuss how they felt it went, what they found useful, and any additional strategies that might help.

Keep the language positive. Whereas sometimes opportunities for patients with a fear of aversive consequences to eat are called exposures by the medical team, using words such as "practice" and doing things "step-by-step" can be more facilitatory in creating a comfortable environment for progress and transformation. Any dietary observations, such as the patient benefiting from a drink but not receiving one or being given a food item they dislike, should be communicated to help improve the next eating opportunity. These strategies, when consistently applied, can significantly enhance the patient's comfort and willingness to engage in the therapeutic process with the occupational therapist.

Assessing and Tracking Progress in Feeding Patterns

- **Observe Eating Patterns**: Eat with the patient to determine their feeding patterns.
- **Document Baseline Data**: Record the patient's baseline behavior and any areas impacting feeding.
- **Monitor Improvements**: Note any changes with therapeutic interventions.

The following charts provide insights into common feeding issues.

By documenting and tracking these issues, therapists can tailor interventions to support each patient's unique needs.

Table 7.1 content covers observations and recommendations for improving eating posture. Video 7.11 reinforces information about optimal mealtime posture:

Table 7.1 Examining physiological patterns and tendencies as they relate to feeding and intake

Posture	Observations	Clinical notes and recommendations
Sitting upright	Patient sits with an upright posture	Maintain as is. An upright posture supports optimal swallowing and breath patterns [40]
Slouching/ Core support	Patient exhibits slouching and lacks core support	Investigate potential causes such as discomfort or lack of core strength. Encourage an ergonomic seating position. Place a pillow or towel rolls behind the back to support improved posture. Consider exercises to strengthen core muscles
Slouched posture due to looking at an iPhone during meals	Patient leans forward and down, often watching an iPhone on the table, resulting in a slouched position and neck strain [41]	For patients who benefit from watching while eating, ensure the device is at or above eye level. Use a stand or elevated item for iPhones, and elevate computers to eye level place a pillow or a pillow roll behind the patient's back to support proper posture. Consider incorporating stretches or strengthening exercises to gradually improve posture. Continue working on posture improvement or consider a referral to physical therapy for further evaluation and treatment
Leaning on table	Patient leans on the table	Determine if this is habitual or occasional. Explore reasons such as fatigue, lack of core strength, or anxiety. Provide support or alternatives
Brings knee(s) to chest while eating	Knee to chest pushes on stomach, though patient may find it comforting, it often results in decreased intake	*Initial observation:* If observed during the meal for the first time, gently recommend relaxing the knees to support eating. If the patient is unable to follow the recommendation, simply observe without further input that meal *Between meal sessions:* • Provide education about the benefits of maintaining a relaxed posture while eating and after eating • If the patient has a fear of vomiting, educate them on why this position is not conducive to abdominal breathing and maintaining a loose body posture • Bringing a knee (or knees) to the chest is often a physiological habit that takes time to shift. Provide ongoing education and opportunities to practice a relaxed seated position during and after eating. • Reinforce the practice of a relaxed seated position with legs relaxed. Criss cross position can work for some patients • Sometimes, patients benefit from sensory input at their feet to avoid bringing the knee to the chest. Consider using a sensory cushion or unpopped plastic hot packs or ice packs at the feet to address this
Chair adjustment	Patient's chair height does not support good posture	Adjust the height and position of the chair to ensure feet are flat on the floor and hips and knees are at 90-degree angles
Back support	Inadequate back support, causing the patient to lean	Use chairs with proper back support or provide additional cushioning. Encourage the patient to sit upright
Feet position	Feet are not flat on the floor, leading to instability	Ensure the patient's feet are flat on the floor or use a footrest (Figs. 7.5 and 7.6). This helps in maintaining an overall good posture

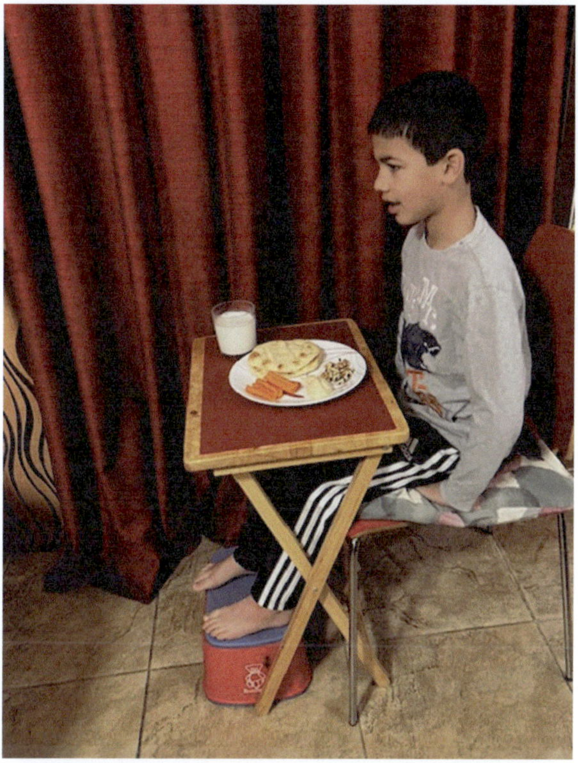

Fig. 7.5 Sitting with postural support of feet supported on a stool and cushioning to raise height so hands easily reach the table

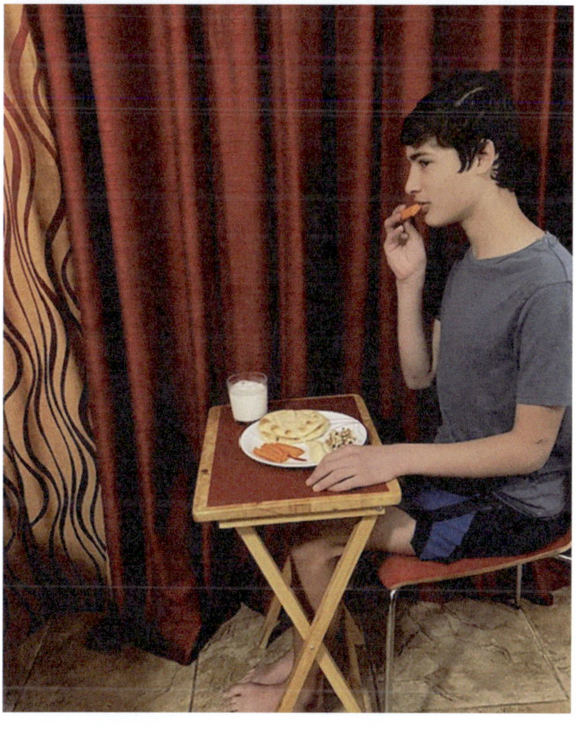

Fig. 7.6 Individual Sitting with relaxed and upright posture where feet touch the floor

Video 7.11 Mealtime Posture Recommendations

https://youtu.be/ZfDwhvDYUJA

QR:

Table 7.2 covers physiological issues that may arise due to fear issues.

Table 7.2 Addressing fear or anxiety based postural issues

Fear or anxiety based postural issues	Observations	Clinical notes and recommendations
Patient muscular tightness at mealtime	Pt elevating shoulders during meal, demonstrating rigidity	Teach the importance of maintaining a loose body posture and the impact of rigidity on the body. The patient may benefit from a pillow behind their back and a stool for their feet if their feet do not reach the ground. Ensure that their food is at arm level and not too high; if necessary, elevate the chair or place cushions/blankets on the chair to achieve better positioning. See (Fig. 7.5)
Reported throat tightness	Chin tuck or observed tightness in neck muscles while eating	Have the patient practice speaking to ensure their vocal quality is clear. It is not uncommon for individuals to complain of throat tightness or demonstrate a physiological pattern that increases tension in their neck or throat. Carefully examine their eating patterns. If they exhibit chin tucking or a tendency to tense their neck or shoulders, provide education on maintaining a neutral, relaxed posture. Encourage practicing this posture between meals and during meals (Video 7.12). Further information in Appendix H.

Video 7.12 Mealtime check-in for optimal position when concerned about a fear of choking

https://youtu.be/WYaHs_5F654

QR:

There are times when issues may arise regarding a patient's fluid intake. These are a high priority if the patient is outpatient as dehydration can result in hospitalization. These also can be addressed within a hospital setting (Table 7.3).

Table 7.3 Drinking patterns: strategies for managing fluid intake during and outside of meals

Drinking pattern	Observations	Clinical notes and recommendations
Drinks water extensively during the meals	Observe if fluid intake seems to be interfering with food intake.	If water consumption does interfere with caloric intake encourage the patient to consume a caloric drink such as milk or juice instead of water during meals. If fluid intake is still interfering with food consumption, encourage smaller sips and decreased frequency of sips
Medical team reports the hospitalized patient is dehydrated.	Pt barely drinking or eating	If a patient is hospitalized and eating and drinking are impacted, occupational therapy focuses on eating first. The medical team will consider whether an IV is required for hydration and will determine the timeline for if an NG is required. Often there is some time to work on feeding prior to an NG requirement
Medical team reports the patient is dehydrated.	Pt barely drinking during or outside of meals.	Have a caloric drink available during meals. If eating is stable or improving, consider a hydration chart (see Chap. 22 Clinical Tools and Protocols appendix I) or application that reinforces achieving the medically requested fluid minimum. Occupational therapists can conduct sessions focusing on improving hydration at set times between meals. Setting a goal about the amount of water or fluid to achieve within the session that includes a set amount of time can be helpful (see Chap. 22 Clinical Tools and Protocols sample hydration pacing appendix J). Use of timers, such as time timers or timers with bell intervals set at every 1–2 min (with expectations to take sips then), can help encourage fluid intake.

There are various oral motor and feeding patterns that may arise while working with a patient (Table 7.4).

Table 7.4 Feeding issues and recommendations

Feeding issue	Reason it may be occuring	Clinical notes and recommendations
Chews exclusively on one side	Developmentally, the patient may not have learned to chew on both sides of the mouth	Teach NUK brush exercises to improve oral motor skills and awareness. Encourage engaging the tongue through this training, followed by consciously practicing chewing on different sides in subsequent meal sessions while referring to NUK brush practice. See further details in NUK brush exercises section
Chews exclusively on one side	Physical factors such as tight braces (current or past), cavities, or other dental issues may contribute to this pattern	Address any necessary corrective dental work if applicable. For issues related to residual patterns from past conditions, use NUK brush exercises and practice to promote bilateral chewing
Report feeling like something is stuck in the throat	Patient may sometime touch the throat or report discomfort but is still able to speak	Have the patient practice speaking, make sure that their vocal quality is clear. If unclear, recommend a bedside swallow evaluation to document observations. If medical causes for throat tightness have not been ruled out, refer for appropriate assessment and continue treatment after. Some patients may experience throat tightening or discomfort when medical causes have been ruled out or treated. Research suggests that carbonated drinks can influence taste receptacles and neuromotor responses [42]. This may help decrease swallow discomfort and improve eating. If this is the case and vocal quality remains clear, keep some carbonated drinks available for the patient to use as needed. Patients may find these drinks helpful with certain foods and tend not to consistently need carbonated drinks
Reported feeling of throat being internally too tight	Patient prefers softer foods	Obtain a referral for a bedside swallow study and document observations. Consult with the medical team and consider a referral for an endoscopy to rule out underlying causes for throat tightness. If the endoscopy results are negative, consider a trial of carbonation as previously mentioned. Examine neck patterns closely to identify or rule out any patterns of neck tightening that may affect swallowing comfort

Feeding

There are methods that can assist patients with improving feeding patterns that are impeding adequate nutrition (Table 7.5).

Table 7.5 Feeding issues and treatment

Issue	Presentation	Treatment
Patient microbiting	Patient takes very small bites of food. This can occur with ARFID- fear patients but sometimes is also present in ARFID-low interest patients	If microbiting occurs with all foods, work with the patient in a structured manner to trial larger bites. Assist them in exploring how to physically manage a larger bolus in their mouth. NUK brush training may benefit these patients. Practicing gum chewing and managing gum boluses can also help
Patient with low tone impacting feeding	Patient with lower muscle tone may also have less physical strength for chewing [43] Assess chewing strength with NUK brush	If an adolescent's baseline tone is low, the OT can work on strengthening exercises with the NUK brush (similar to the exercises mentioned above) away from meal times to avoid fatigue. Linking these exercises to times when the patient brushes their teeth, such as upon waking and before sleep, can be effective. If the patient has very low tone or is unable to improve oral motor strength, consider carefully choosing their diet to avoid large quantities of very crunchy foods (e.g., raw vegetables). Recognize that some supplementation and nutritional drinks (e.g., milk, juices, or meals with supplements served simultaneously) may be necessary. Children with lower tone often benefit from eating softer foods first. If there is a crunchy or chewier food, target it last, and then if further nutrition is needed, use a supplement or drink to meet the full caloric needs of that meal. Help the patient understand their strengths and challenges and what can make eating easier for them
Immature munching pattern	Patient chews food in up-and-down pattern without a rotary chew	Implement NUK brush exercises. Ensure there is no tongue tie present. Additionally, consider incorporating mewing gum exercises to better engage the tongue with large gum boluses

(continued)

Table 7.5 (continued)

Issue	Presentation	Treatment
Struggles with mid-range textures (e.g., rice with lentils, certain softer pastas)	Chews mid-range textures for a long time. May hold them in the cheek	Alternate between mid-range textures and crunchier foods that provide more sensory input to the mouth (e.g., chips, crunchy carrots). This input helps improve the chewing process. Encourage the patient to take a bite of a crunchier food while still chewing the mid-range texture to increase sensory input. This will either elicit a swallow or improved chewing. Emphasize the importance of moving food to the opposite side of the mouth. Encourage the patient to apply the skills learned from NUK brush exercises during meals by chewing for 10 times, moving the food bolus to the opposite side, repeating if needed, and then swallowing. Occasionally, the patient may need to show the therapist the food (by opening their mouth) to ensure it is ready to swallow. Difficulty swallowing mid-range textures is typically due to not fully interpreting the texture and not fully engaging the tongue in eating (Video 7.13)
Struggling with thicker texture of a food, like peanut butter	Reports throat feeling uncomfortable, slowing down	Alternate food bites with another food. Make a drink or other item available that changes the input to the mouth

Video 7.13 Tips for Picky Eaters

https://youtu.be/D96DAieizb8

QR:

It is important to know what strategies may assist the patient, to teach them between the meal periods and to support utilizing them during a meal [Table 7.6].

Table 7.6 Monitoring patient presentation and addressing issues during meals

Issue	Presentation	Treatment
Is not demonstrating the ability to get enough food to meet caloric needs	Early satiety	Utilize pressure points to help manage feelings of fullness. Implement gradual, step-by-step increases in food intake each day (or every couple of days) to help the individual get accustomed to more nutrition. Ensure that food increases are step-by-step and do not exceed a 100 kcal increase per day unless initiated by the patient. Provide the opportunity for more intake without making it a requirement Develop the skill of consuming a small amount of supplement at each meal and snack. Start with an amount that can be completed each time and gradually build up to 2 oz. at each meal and snack Once the patient is consistently consuming 1000+ kcals and able to take 2 oz. of supplement at each meal and snack, implement a ladder block plan or eat-replace plan. Gradually increase the ladder block kcals or eatreplace kcals until the patient reaches the goal set by the RD
Picky eater	Rejects trials of new foods or foods they once liked and have jagged out on	Utilize a food exploration log (refer to form and details below) Introduce newer or previously consumed foods at the beginning of the meal Rotate in foods that are rated "like it" 3 or higher with the food exploration log, always presenting them at the start of the meal Gradually increase the expected quantity as the patient becomes more comfortable taking bites If the patient is not internally motivated to try new foods, consider implementing a reward based behavior modification plan to encourage this change
Nausea	Demonstrates discomfort while eating and reports nausea	Utilize and reinforce techniques taught for addressing nausea. Assist the patient in using the techniques and determining which ones are helpful
Patient feels concerned that they will vomit	Patient appears nervous and states they will vomit	Reinforce a loose body position. If they have learned abdominal breathing, pause and practice it during the session. If they have not yet learned, return and teach it between sessions.
Patient starts crying	Tearfulness making it difficult for the patient to eat	Have the patient pause eating until tearfulness subsides. Explain that there will be an opportunity to fully express their concerns between meals, but during the meal, it can be helpful to focus on setting the emotion aside to care for the body. Ensure to follow up between meals to discuss strategies if crying arises again. Inform the psych team of the situation

These charts are not all-inclusive. Through activity analysis and ongoing assessment, the occupational therapist can examine barriers that arise during meal times and address them step-by-step, enabling the patient to reach their highest functional level.

Productive Coping Strategies List

One of the key features of treating ARFID is building the skill of using productive coping strategies. It is important to brainstorm and have the patient document these strategies as they are taught by various team members. Encouraging patients to teach the coping strategies they learn to family members or friends, either in person or through a virtual meeting platform, will further engage their ability to use and remember these strategies. Coping strategies lists can be made and categorized in a variety of ways. The example below includes three sections:

Wisdom & Inspiration (Things you Tell yourself in Moments of Challenge)

To elicit useful statements, ask questions such as, "What do you tell yourself if you have homework that you are not in the mood to do?" or "What do you tell yourself when something is challenging to learn in a sport or other activity?" These statements, which the patient has found helpful in overcoming challenges, can be extended to the challenging situations they face while expanding their foods or coping with sensations.

Action Strategies (Things that Shift Sensations or Feelings)

Most of the strategies to address barriers fall under this category. These are practical actions that help manage sensations or feelings effectively.

Distraction Strategies (Taking the Mind off Sensations or Feelings for a Period of Time)

Distraction strategies help divert attention away from discomfort. For example, watching a great movie can temporarily take someone's mind off pain, and they may notice that the pain has faded or bothers them less after the movie ends. Examples could include doing artwork or talking to a friend.

> **Sample Coping Strategies**
> The below Productive Coping Strategies chart [Fig. 7.7] was developed with a patient.. Some of these strategies (e.g., abdominal breathing with loose body posture, use of a hot pack) were taught at the eval and others were developed and documented at subsequent sessions.

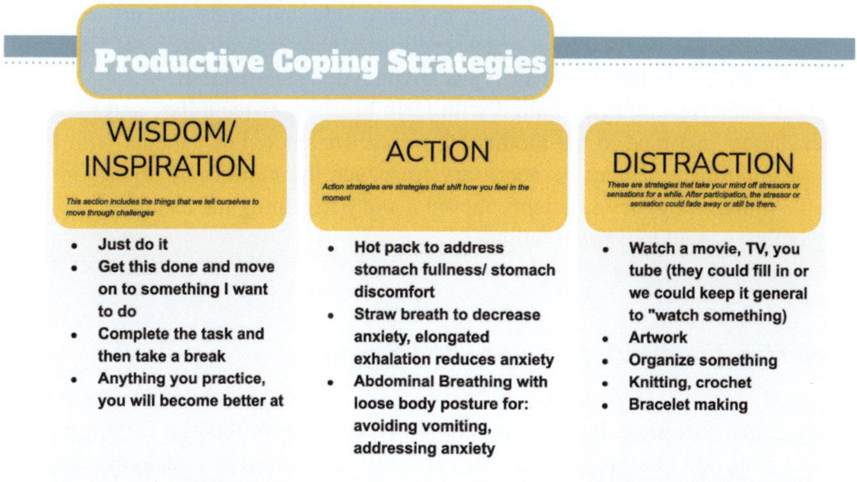

Fig. 7.7 Sample Productive Coping Strategy chart for an individual with anxiety and a fear of vomiting

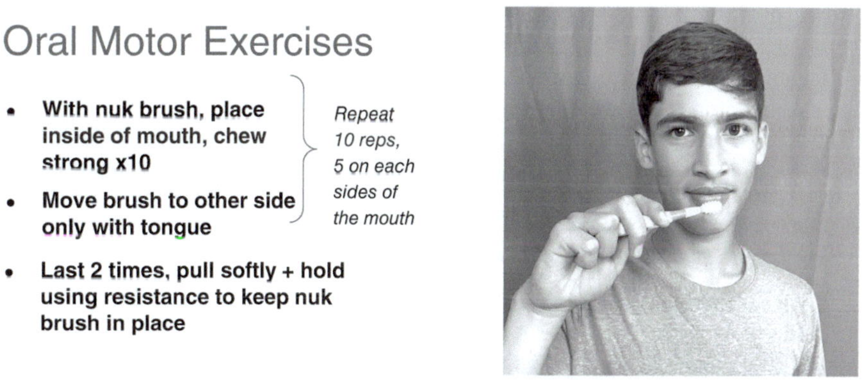

Fig. 7.8 NUK Brush exercises (full-size available in Chap. 22 Appendix N)

NUK Brush Exercises

NUK brush exercises benefit a variety of ARFID patients: ARFID patients that tend to chew only on one side by habit or due to a prior pain issue (e.g., previously tight braces, cavity), ARFID patients with a fear of aversive consequences who have built developed a habit of barely chewing, patients with oral motor delays who can benefit from improved tongue use and chewing patterns.

NUK Brush Exercises (Fig. 7.8) serve as both an initial tool for examining oral motor strength and tongue movement, and as a method to encourage improved chewing. Instruct the patient to chew the brush on one side for 10 chews, then use their tongue to move the brush to the opposite side and repeat the process. This sequence can be done for a total of 10 repetitions, with repetitions 9 and 10 including a bite and gentle pull to enhance jaw strength and stabilization.

These exercises are often paired with teeth brushing twice a day, and the NUK brush can be kept next to the toothbrush for convenience. For patients with lower tone or endurance, it may be necessary to reduce the number of repetitions and chews. Additionally, these patients should avoid performing the exercises immediately before a meal to prevent fatigue.

Exploring Food with Structure and Support

Occupational therapists have been supporting youth with feeding difficulties for decades [44], long before ARFID was officially recognized as a diagnosis. Across various professional realms, numerous methods and structures have been developed to aid in the intake of newer or previously eliminated foods.

One such tool is the Step-by-Step Food Exploration Log ([Fig. 7.9] and full-size available in Chap. 22, Appendix N Worksheet Section), created by Anne Sinha in 2016. This log, also known simply as the Food Exploration Log, is designed to support patients in scientifically testing out foods in a structured and supportive manner.

Patients with ARFID, particularly those with a sensory subtype, often benefit from using a food exploration journal (Video 7.14) (see additional RD-created Trial Tracker in Chap. 22, Appendix 5). Additionally, the log can be valuable for those who fear aversive consequences and are hesitant to retry previously tolerated foods, offering a safe and structured way to reintroduce them.

Video 7.14 Use of the Step-by-Step Food Exploration Log

https://youtu.be/QAkMLqtRfLg

The log can also be useful when taste testing different supplements that may be used as a replacement or to supplement nutrition. Often anywhere from two to five different supplement types and flavors can be tested. Patients tend to do better with choice and options, so this allows a neutral way to taste test and once their taste test is completed, The patient can be asked to rank the favored supplement in numeric order.

Directions for Food Exploration Log: (Record all answers on log, when possible, staff or family should fill out the log so that the patient can focus on eating).
- Prior to starting, patient's food to be explored and preferred change-taste food/drink and a drink should be in front of them. Review what change-taste taste food item is (i.e., an enjoyed item to change the flavor of the food).
- Newer foods should be trialed at the start of the meal, prior to any other item.
- Have individual with ARFID first rank appearance prior to taking a bite. 0= looks terrible, 5= looks great, 3= in the middle.
- Review that the first bite will be to rank texture, 0-5, 0= terrible texture, 5= great texture, 3= in the middle.
- Let them know the next bite is a ranking of flavor. 0= terrible flavor, 5= great flavor, 3 = in the middle.
- Let them know the next bite is for ranking "like it." 0= do not like it at all, 5= like it a lot, 3= in the middle.
- Ask, do you think you would try it again on another day? Yes, No, Maaaybe? It's good to extend the maybe out as it often helps them consider it more. If they disliked it, consider saying, "Do you think you would try it in a different form (e.g., crunchier, more cooked, with a dip, etc.)?"
- If the food has been trialed before, indicate how many times in "Trial of this Food #."

Step-by-Step Food Exploration Log

(to support growth, health, energy and a full life)

Please have at least 3 bites of a newer food at meals and/or snacks and rank 1- 5 below. Take a bite to explore texture, a bite to explore flavor and a bite to explore "like it."

Date	Item Name	Appearance 0-5	Texture 0-5	Flavor 0-5	Like it 0-5	Do you think you try it again on a different day? (Yes, no, maybe)	Quantity eaten:	Trial of this Food #

Fig. 7.9 Food exploration log

Step-by-Step Food Exploration Log

Once a relationship is established with the patient and they are getting enough nutrition to stay medically stable, it is worthwhile to consider use of the Food Exploration Log in subsequent sessions. When introducing the food exploration log, explain to patients that the goal is to examine and experience the food "as a scientist would." A scientist conducts experiments with a "layer of neutrality," allowing for an unbiased examination of observations.

Preparation Steps:

1. **Establish a "Changeover" Food or Drink (see Chap. 5 Nutrition):**
   - Identify a favored food or drink that the patient will have available, as needed, to follow less-preferred flavors.
   - A preferred crunchy food can also provide helpful chewing input
   - Allow the patient to choose their "changeover" food, which might be a chip, candy, sweet, or preferred drink.
   - Review with the patient that the newer food should not be spit out during the trial. Instead, they can change the flavor by consuming a known and enjoyed food immediately after the trial bite.
2. **Timing of the Food Exploration Log:**
   - Conduct the log at the start of a regular meal or snack when the patient is likely to be hungry.
   - This encourages the patient to try and potentially accept the new food as part of their meal.
3. **Consider what food to taste test:** Table 7.7 can be referenced to determine what foods to explore and the priority level based on patient presentation.

Using the Food Exploration Log:

1. **Introduce the Log:**
   - Explain the concept of experiencing the food "as a scientist would."
   - Briefly discuss the medicinal or valuable qualities of the food (e.g., carrots have vitamin A, tofu has protein, pizza is a common party food).
2. **Step-by-Step Process:**
   - **Visual Examination and Ranking:** Have the patient look at the food and rank it from 1–5 (1 = terrible, 5 = great, 3 = in the middle).
   - **Texture Evaluation:** Ask the patient to take a bite and rank the texture based on their preference.
   - **Flavor Evaluation:** Have them take another bite and rank the flavor.
   - **Overall Preference:** Finally, ask them to take another bite and rank their overall liking of the food.

Table 7.7 Foods to add in priority and consideration

Issue	Priority to trial with food exploration log	Priority level
Low weight	Previously consumed calorically dense foods	High
Low weight	New dense foods that the family cooks/ has available on a regular basis	Medium high
Vitamin or nutrient deficiency	Foods that will enable the meeting of the missing nutrient, brainstorm all with RD input and pick with patient	High
Has few foods in their food rotation	Previously consumed foods	High
Has few foods in their food rotation	Food that expands their food intake types (e.g., a protein or dairy food if they only eat carbs) that the family cooks/ has available on a regular basis. Take RD input	Medium-high
Patient's weight is within normal limits but there are whole food groups that they do not eat	Food that expands their food intake types (e.g., a vegetable, fruit or fruit juice if they don't have any) that the family cooks/ has available on a regular basis	Medium
Patient is able to get enough food at home but struggles to get nutrition when traveling or when at a friend's house	Bites of food that would be available at a restaurant (consider the type of restaurants family members go to) or friend's house	High-medium
Patient is able to get enough food at home but struggles with food outside of the house and is leaving for college within a year	Portions of foods that will be readily available at college. Once practice occurs prioritize going to cafeterias to practice further	High
Patient will be going on a trip (school or other) and often does not eat enough outside of the house	Determine what will be served in area they are going to, replicate and practice food exploration with similar foods	High

3. **Handling Hesitation:**
   - Allow the patient to choose the bite size. If they hesitate, reassure them by reminding them that they choose the bite size and about the "change-taste" food.

4. **Follow-Up:**
   - If the ranking for the food item "liking it" is 3 or above, ask if they can try the food again on another day.
   - If the ranking is 2–3 (different patients are more conservative with their 3 s, so sometimes 3 represents a dislike whereas for others it is "okay" or "new.") ask if they can try the food again and under different conditions (e.g., cooked differently, with a dip).
   - If rankings is a 1, do not assign that as a try food.

5. **Parental Involvement:**
   - If the patient agrees to try the food again, work with parents to present the food at least three times in the following week at the start of meals or snacks.
   - Ensure these opportunities occur during low-pressure times of day.

6. **Rewards:**

   - Depending on the patient's age and level of intrinsic motivation, incorporating rewards for participating in the food exploration can be beneficial.
   - Rewards can be integrated into a larger behavior modification plan, such as earning points, or provided as immediate incentives for each food exploration.
   - For some patients, offering a choice of their favored food while trying the food exploration item can also serve as an inherent reward.

Regular use of the food exploration log is recommended, even when revisiting the same foods at home without the occupational therapist. Over time, patients can record the number of times they have tried a food beside it rather than re-ranking repeat tries. As the food becomes more accepted, gradually increasing the quantity until it is regularly incorporated into meals is advised. Food exploration and expansion take time, but any new food added to a sensory eater's diet can be highly valuable. Parent involvement is essential, as food exploration cannot succeed without it. Often, getting parents to present the foods regularly at the start of a meal is one of the most significant steps and sometimes obstacles in helping the patient develop the skill of food expansion.

Supporting patients with ARFID in making meaningful changes to their eating patterns, quantity, and food variety requires a comprehensive and hands-on approach. By actively participating in meals with the patients, occupational therapists and speech therapists can provide real-time observation and intervention, which is instrumental for identifying and addressing specific barriers to eating. This approach not only allows therapists to offer immediate support and encouragement but also helps in modeling positive eating behaviors and establishing a comfortable and supportive environment.

The strategies outlined in this section, including the use of food exploration logs, productive coping strategies, and maintaining a neutral and pleasant atmosphere during meals, are essential tools in the therapeutic process. By integrating these approaches, therapists can foster a sense of safety and trust, encouraging patients to gradually expand their dietary repertoire and improve their overall intake.

Ultimately, the goal is to empower patients to overcome their challenges with eating and enhancing their quality of life. Consistent, empathetic, and informed support from occupational therapists can make a significant difference in the progress and success of patients with ARFID.

References

1. Stern RM, Koch KL, Andrews PLR. Nausea: mechanisms and management. Oxford University Press; 2011. https://lane.stanford.edu/view/sul/12940554
2. Nelwati N, Noviyani D. The effect of diaphragmatic breathing on nausea, vomiting and functional status among breast cancer patients undergoing chemotherapy. Eur J Oncol Nurs. 2024;70:102548. Lee A, Fan, LT (2009) Stimulation of the wrist acupuncture point P6 for preventing postoperative nausea and vomiting. *The Cochrane database of systematic reviews*, (2), CD003281. https://doi.org/10.1002/14651858.CD003281.pub3.
3. Grossmann I, Sahdra BK, Ciarrochi J. A heart and A mind: self-distancing facilitates the association between heart rate variability, and wise reasoning. Front Behav Neurosci. 2016;10:68. https://doi-org.laneproxy.stanford.edu/10.3389/fnbeh.2016.00068
4. Lee A, Fan LT. Stimulation of the wrist acupuncture point P6 for preventing postoperative nausea and vomiting. Cochrane Database Syst Rev. 2009;2:CD003281. https://doi.org/10.1002/14651858.CD003281.pub3.
5. Steele NM, French J, Gatherer-Boyles J, Newman S, Leclaire S. Effect of acupressure by sea-bands on nausea and vomiting of pregnancy. J Obst Gyne Neonatal Nursing: JOGNN. 2001;30(1):61–70. https://lane.stanford.edu/view/pubmed/11277163
6. White PF, Issioui T, Hu J, Jones SB, Coleman JE, Waddle JP, Markowitz SD, Coloma M, Macaluso AR, Ing CH. Comparative efficacy of acustimulation (ReliefBand) versus ondansetron (Zofran) in combination with droperidol for preventing nausea and vomiting. Anesthesiology. 2002;97(5):1075–81. https://doi-org.laneproxy.stanford.edu/10.1097/00000542-200211000-00008
7. Asay K, Olson C, Donnelly J, Perlman E. The use of aromatherapy in postoperative nausea and vomiting: A systematic review. J Perianesthesia Nursing: Off J American Soc of PeriAnesthesia Nurses. 2019;34(3):502–16. https://doi-org.laneproxy.stanford.edu/10.1016/j.jopan.2018.08.006
8. Spencer KW. Isopropyl alcohol inhalation as treatment for nausea and vomiting. Plastic Sur Nursing: Official J American Soc Plastic Reconstruct Sur Nurses. 2004;24(4):149–54. https://doi-org.laneproxy.stanford.edu/10.1097/00006527-200410000-00005
9. Ernst E, Pittler MH. Efficacy of ginger for nausea and vomiting: a systematic review of randomized clinical trials. Br J Anaesth. 2000;84(3):367–71. https://doi-org.laneproxy.stanford.edu/10.1093/oxfordjournals.bja.a013442
10. Wazqar D, Thabet H, Safwat A. A quasi-experimental study of the effect of ginger tea on preventing nausea and vomiting in patients with gynecological cancers receiving cisplatin-based regimens. Cancer Nurs. 2021;44(6):E513–9. https://doi.org/10.1097/NCC.0000000000000939.
11. Iwata G, Iwai N, Nagashima M, Fukata R. New biofeedback therapy in children with encopresis. European J Pediat Surgery: off J Austrian Assoc Pediatric Sur … [et al] = Zeitschrift fur Kinderchirurgie. 1995;5(4):231–4. https://doi-org.laneproxy.stanford.edu/10.1055/s-2008-1066212
12. Kaatz D. Characters of wisdom: Taoist tales of the acupuncture points [Kindle edition]. The Petite Bergerie Press; 2011.
13. Asadi N, Maharlouei N, Khalili A, Darabi Y, Davoodi S, Raeisi Shahraki H, Hadianfard M, Jokar A, Vafaei H, Kasraeian M. Effects of LI-4 and SP-6 acupuncture on labor pain, cortisol level and duration of labor. J Acupunct Meridian Stud. 2015;8(5):249–54. https://doi-org.laneproxy.stanford.edu/10.1016/j.jams.2015.08.003
14. Chilman LB, Meredith PJ, Southon N, Kennedy-Behr A, Frakking T, Swanepoel L, Verdonck M. Occupational performance coaching for parents of picky eaters: A mixed methods study. Aust Occup Ther J. 2024; https://doi.org/10.1111/1440-1630.12947. Advance online publication. https://doi-org.laneproxy.stanford.edu/10.1111/1440-1630.12947
15. Petell JA, Bilsky SA. An examination of the association between emotion regulation and Emetophobia symptoms. Psychol Rep. 2023;332941231213855. Advance online publication. https://doi-org.laneproxy.stanford.edu/10.1177/00332941231213855

16. Heaton-Harris N. Living with emetophobia: coping with extreme fear of vomiting. Jessica Kingsley Publishers; 2007. p. 129. https://lane.stanford.edu/view/sul/12994828
17. Halland M, Parthasarathy G, Bharucha AE, Katzka DA. Diaphragmatic breathing for rumination syndrome: efficacy and mechanisms of action. Neurogastroenterol Motil. 2016;28(3):384–91. https://doi-org.laneproxy.stanford.edu/10.1111/nmo.12737
18. Robles A, Romero YA, Tatro E, Quezada H, McCallum RW. Outcomes of treating rumination syndrome with a tricyclic antidepressant and diaphragmatic breathing. Am J Med Sci. 2020;360(1):42–9. https://doi-org.laneproxy.stanford.edu/10.1016/j.amjms.2020.04.003
19. Subbalakshmi NK, Adhikari P, Shanmugavel Jeganathan P. Comparative study on cardiac autonomic modulation during deep breathing test and diaphragmatic breathing in type 2 diabetes and healthy subjects. J Diabetes Invest. 2014;5(4):456–63.
20. Mosa HES, El-Bready HG, El-Sol AEH, Bayomy HE, Taman RO, Shehata HS. Efficacy of abdominal breathing on sleep and quality of life among patients with non-erosive gastroesophageal reflux. J Public Health Res. 2024;13(1):22799036241231788. https://doi-org.laneproxy.stanford.edu/10.1177/22799036241231788
21. Chitkara DK, Van Tilburg M, Whitehead WE, Talley NJ. Teaching diaphragmatic breathing for rumination syndrome. Am J Gastroenterol. 2006;101(11):2449–52. https://doi-org.laneproxy.stanford.edu/10.1111/j.1572-0241.2006.00801.x
22. Feillet, F., Bocquet, A., Briend, A., Chouraqui, J. P., Darmaun, D., Frelut, M. L., Girardet, J. P., Guimber, D., Hankard, R., Lapillonne, A., Peretti, N., Rozé, J. C., Simeoni, U., Turck, D., Dupont, C., & Comité de nutrition de la Société française de pédiatrie (CNSFP) (2019). Nutritional risks of ARFID (avoidant restrictive food intake disorders) and related behavior. Archives de pediatrie: organe officiel de la Societe francaise de pediatrie, 26(7), 437–441. https://doi-org.laneproxy.stanford.edu/10.1016/j.arcped.2019.08.005.
23. Mutyala R, Sanders K, Bates MD. Assessment and management of pediatric constipation for the primary care clinician. Curr Probl Pediatr Adolesc Health Care. 2020;50(5):100802. https://doi-org.laneproxy.stanford.edu/10.1016/j.cppeds.2020.100802
24. Mattheus HK, Wagner C, Becker K, Bühren K, Correll CU, Egberts KM, Ehrlich S, Fleischhaker C, Föcker M, Hahn F, Hebebrand J, Herpertz-Dahlmann B, Jaite C, Jenetzky E, Kaess M, Legenbauer PD, T., Pfeiffer PhD, J. P., Renner Md, T. J., Roessner, V., Schulze, U., … von Gontard, A. Incontinence and constipation in adolescent patients with anorexia nervosa-results of a multicenter study from a German web-based registry for children and adolescents with anorexia nervosa. Int J Eat Disord. 2020;53(2):219–28. https://doi-org.laneproxy.stanford.edu/10.1002/eat.23182
25. Bolia R, Safe M, Southwell BR, King SK, Oliver MR. Paediatric constipation for general paediatricians: review using a case-based and evidence-based approach. J Paediatr Child Health. 2020;56(11):1708–18. https://doi-org.laneproxy.stanford.edu/10.1111/jpc.14720
26. Harvey S, Matthai S, King DA. How to use the Bristol stool chart in childhood constipation. *Archives of disease in childhood*. Educ Pract Edition. 2023;108(5):335–9. https://doi-org.laneproxy.stanford.edu/10.1136/archdischild-2022-324513
27. Modi RM, Hinton A, Pinkhas D, Groce R, Meyer MM, Balasubramanian G, Levine E, Stanich PP. Implementation of a defecation posture modification device: impact on bowel movement patterns in healthy subjects. J Clin Gastroenterol. 2019;53(3):216–9. https://doi-org.laneproxy.stanford.edu/10.1097/MCG.0000000000001143
28. Thomas JJ, Brigham KS, Sally ST, Hazen EP, Eddy KT. Case 18-2017 – an 11-year-old girl with difficulty eating after a choking incident. N Engl J Med. 2017;376(24):2377–86. https://doi-org.laneproxy.stanford.edu/10.1056/NEJMcpc1616394
29. McNally RJ. Choking phobia: a review of the literature. Compr Psychiatry. 1994;35(1):83–9. https://doi-org.laneproxy.stanford.edu/10.1016/0010-440x(94)90174-0
30. Begotka A, Silverman A, Goday P. Protocolized intervention for children and adolescents with Phagophobia. J Pediatr Gastroenterol Nutr. 2022;75(6):e107–10. https://doi-org.laneproxy.stanford.edu/10.1097/MPG.0000000000003628

31. McClain BC, Suresh S, editors. Handbook of pediatric chronic pain: current science and integrative practice. Springer; 2011. https://lane.stanford.edu/view/bib/297906
32. Goodall J, Brown T. Patients' experiences of occupational therapy within a multidisciplinary pain management programme: A qualitative study. Br J Pain. 2022;16(3):290–302. https://doi.org/10.1177/20494637211054697.
33. Marcus DA. Chronic pain: A primary care guide to practical management. 2nd ed. Humana Press; 2009. https://lane.stanford.edu/view/sul/13365157
34. Chesney, A. B., & Brorsen, N. E. (2000). OT's role in managing chronic pain. OT Practice.. https://communot.aota.org/viewdocument/18-october-9-2000
35. Boradyn KM, Przybyłowicz KE, Jarocka-Cyrta E. Low FODMAP diet is not effective in children with functional abdominal pain: A randomized controlled trial. Ann Nutr Metab. 2020;76(5):334–44. https://doi-org.laneproxy.stanford.edu/10.1159/000510795
36. Zickgraf HF, Loftus P, Gibbons B, Cohen LC, Hunt MG. "if I could survive without eating, it would be a huge relief": development and initial validation of the fear of food questionnaire. Appetite. 2022;169:105808. https://doi-org.laneproxy.stanford.edu/10.1016/j.appet.2021.105808
37. Fitzgerald M, Frankum B. Food avoidance and restriction in adults: a cross-sectional pilot study comparing patients from an immunology clinic to a general practice. J Eat Disord. 2017;5:30. https://doi.org/10.1186/s40337-017-0160-4.
38. Min KC, Seo SM, Woo HS. Effect of oral motor facilitation technique on oral motor and feeding skills in children with cerebral palsy: a case study. BMC Pediatr. 2022;22(1):626. https://doi.org/10.1186/s12887-022-03674-8.
39. Reche-Olmedo L, Torres-Collado L, Compañ-Gabucio LM, Garcia-de-la-Hera M. The role of occupational therapy in managing food selectivity of children with autism Spectrum disorder: A scoping review. Children (Basel, Switzerland). 2021;8(11):1024. https://doi.org/10.3390/children8111024.
40. Yoshikawa M, Nagakawa K, Tanaka R, Yamawaki K, Mori T, Hiraoka A, Higa C, Nishikawa Y, Yoshida M, Tsuga K. Improper sitting posture while eating adversely affects maximum tongue pressure. J Dental Sci. 2021;16(1):467–73. https://doi-org.laneproxy.stanford.edu/10.1016/j.jds.2020.08.012
41. Tegtmeier P. A scoping review on smart mobile devices and physical strain. Work (Reading, Mass). 2018;59(2):273–83. https://doi-org.laneproxy.stanford.edu/10.3233/WOR-172678
42. Moritaka H, Kitade M, Sawamura S, Takihara T, Awano I, Ono T, Tamine K, Hori K. Effect of carbon dioxide in carbonated drinks on linguapalatal swallowing pressure. Chem Senses. 2014;39(2):133–42. https://doi-org.laneproxy.stanford.edu/10.1093/chemse/bjt062
43. Sarnat HB. Neuromuscular disorders. In: Behrman RE, Kliegman RM, Jenson HB, editors. Nelson textbook of pediatrics. 17th ed. Saunders; 2004. p. 2053.
44. Potter P, Harryman S. Physical and occupational therapy for the handicapped child. Pediatr Clin N Am. 1973;20(1):159–76. https://doi-org.laneproxy.stanford.edu/10.1016/s0031-3955(16)32817-6

Chapter 8
Feeding Plans for ARFID Patients

Parent Training

Effective feeding strategies for ARFID patients, particularly those with low weight or experiencing weight loss, benefit from a multidisciplinary approach ideally involving the occupational therapist and other healthcare team members. Central to this approach is the training and support of parents or caregivers to foster an environment that encourages adequate nutrition. Tools such as the Ladder Block Plan, alongside behavior modification strategies, can be incorporated into feeding plans to support both patients and their families. Parents play a crucial role in supporting their child's nutritional intake, and training them to remain present and attentive during meals is essential. The healthcare team can collaborate with the patient and family to develop personalized plans when agreed upon.

A key aspect of training parents is teaching the "layer of neutrality," which involves supporting their child to eat while maintaining a neutral, non-reactive demeanor. Parents should be encouraged to keep mealtime conversations neutral, avoiding potentially stressful topics such as school, family, or politics. Instead, discussions can focus on pleasant subjects like travel, family pets, or light-hearted stories. Some families find that reading a book or engaging in a simple, non-distracting game can help maintain a calm atmosphere during meals. The benefits of family meals are well-documented [1, 2], and creating a positive mealtime environment can support the likelihood of meeting nutritional goals.

Patients with ARFID, across all subtypes, may require more time to consume meals compared to their peers. It is not uncommon for these patients to take up to an hour to complete meals or large snacks. Ensuring that adequate time is allocated for meals, while also fitting within the patient's daily schedule, is essential for their nutritional progress. Caregivers should be prepared to sit with the child throughout the extended mealtime [3] offering support as needed.

A. B. Sinha et al., *Comprehensive Clinical Care for Adolescents with Avoidant/Restrictive Food Intake Disorder (ARFID)*,
https://doi.org/10.1007/978-3-031-92232-9_8

For ARFID patients who are underweight, as well as most growing youth, maintaining regular meal and snack times is important to meet their energetic and cognitive needs. The occupational therapist can support the patient in developing rituals and routines [4, 5] around mealtime. Establishing a routine of three meals and two snacks, such as an after-school snack and a nighttime snack, can support weight gain. Some patients, particularly those with ARFID characterized by low interest in food or fear of aversive consequences, may require additional nutritional opportunities. In these cases, incorporating an extra morning snack into their daily routine may be necessary. Additionally, for younger patients who have an early bedtime, a morning snack can serve as an alternative approach to a nighttime snack.

Digital:Video 8.1 Importance of Eating at Regular Intervals
https://youtu.be/RJmW-oYlxLM

Patients may require guidance to remember to notice and work on their posture [6], breathing patterns, and use of coping strategies [7]. Many benefit from distraction through conversation or, when appropriate, media, provided it does not reduce their intake. Families should choose distractions that align with their personal mealtime preferences and values. For example, if a video is used to provide pleasant distraction, it could be a shared experience where both the youth and the parent can watch together without the use of earbuds. Additionally, participating in a meaningful activity after a meal can be beneficial and help patients cope as they move through their physical and emotional sensations, especially if they feel full or anxious due to fear-related issues.

Establishing a routine of regular food intake is important, particularly for patients focused on weight gain. Incorporating liquid supplements as a calorie-for-calorie replacement for incomplete nutrition or as an add-on to meals to increase caloric intake can be highly beneficial. When full replacement is not feasible, gradually introducing the practice of consistently consuming a small amount of supplement at meals and snacks can be an effective approach to building the skill of using a supplement. Many ARFID patients may benefit from having foods with varying tastes or textures that change the sensory input between bites. Including these foods as part of the meal or making them accessible as add-ons can be advantageous. For patients who experience throat discomfort, having a carbonated beverage available (in the same room but not directly presented during the meal) can be valuable if needed.

The use of a food exploration log, both during and outside of occupational therapy sessions, can be beneficial for patients working on food expansion. Collaborating with parents to ensure that new foods introduced are already available at home or are easily accessible can increase the likelihood of these foods being consistently rotated into meals. Additionally, guiding parents in developing the habit of regularly presenting new (and recently trialed) foods at the beginning of meals or snacks can reinforce this practice. Reward plans or other motivators can be effective in encouraging patient cooperation during the food expansion process.

Educational Accommodations

Supporting the patient and family in fitting meals into their schedule is important. Occupational therapists use temporal adaptation [8] to support fitting meals into the daily activities and routines. For patients who struggle to consume enough food during school hours, adjustments to their meal schedule may be necessary. In some cases, a family member, teaching staff, or school nurse may need to join the youth for lunch. Alternatively, parents may consider shifting the balance between lunch and snacks, providing a larger meal after school when the child may have more time and will be less distracted by the school day.

In a school setting, accommodations may be necessary to support sufficient time for meals. These may include allowing the student to leave class early to enter the lunch line, arrive late to class after finishing lunch, or eat food during class. These accommodations are vital for ensuring their child receives adequate nutrition during the school day. The medical team can provide supporting documentation to advocate for a 504 or individualized education plan when necessary.

Meal/Snack Replacement Approach: The Eat-Replace Model

Please see the nutrition section for a full description of this feeding strategy. When using an eat-replace plan for feeding, the patient consumes what they can of the meal and the missing caloric value is provided through a liquid supplement replacement. When weight gain is a priority, it is important to choose a supplement that is dense in calories in order to get the most value from the supplement. See video 8.2 https://www.youtube.com/watch?v=0b9qGDHRBF0. If the patient cannot immediately do an eat-replace plan, but can build to that point, consider doing it sequentially, as is referenced in Video 8.3 Building the skill of taking a supplement.

Video 8.2 Use of Supplements to support weight gain
https://www.youtube.com/watch?v=0b9qGDHRBF0

There are patterns for priorities in developing feeding plans amongst subtypes:

Low Interest

When working with Low Interest ARFID patients, the first priority is to trial an eat-replace model while reinforcing the importance of schedule, routines and making food a priority. In this model the food needed is presented, whatever is not consumed is replaced with a high-density supplement provided at the meal end. Activity analysis can help with examining the barriers to nutrition. If the eat-replace model is not effective, consider the Ladder Block Plan or a similar program that helps the patients calculate that they are eating enough at regular intervals. Sometimes simple behavior modifications that reinforce food quantity, eating at regular intervals and use of productive coping strategies can also be useful.

Sensory Eater

For sensory eaters, whether in an outpatient or inpatient setting, it is crucial to first assess whether weight is a significant concern. If low weight is an issue, the focus should be on reinforcing adequate nutrition through preferred foods, supplements, and any newly introduced foods to prevent hospitalization and support proper functioning. Implementing the Ladder Block Plan can help establish a routine of consistently consuming enough nutrition.

When managing sensory eaters in an outpatient setting, if weight or weight loss is not a concern, the initial priority may be on reintroducing previously consumed foods. The Food Exploration Log serves as a valuable tool in this process. Patients should be encouraged to practice consuming items ranked as a 3 or higher during food exploration at least three times per week. Families can be supported in developing the skill of having the patient explore new food items independently, gradually incorporating newer foods. Adding a reward component for trying new foods and maintaining them throughout the week can further motivate the patient (see Occupational Therapy-Developed Worksheet Step-by-Step Food Exploration Log with Reward in Chap. 22).

In an inpatient setting, close collaboration with the dietitian (RD) is essential to provide the patient with sufficient vitamins and adequate nutrition. Taste testing of supplements and gradually increasing supplement quantities should be prioritized. Depending on the patient's tolerance, an eat-replace model may be used if the supplement is well-tolerated, or a Ladder Block Plan can be considered if the supplement is accepted in small quantities but is not preferred. Additionally, training in pill swallowing for vitamin intake, trialing newer or previously consumed foods through the Food Exploration Log, and applying the Ladder Block Plan if consistent nutrition intake is not achieved are critical components of the inpatient sensory eater's management plan.

Fear of Aversive Consequences

For patients with a fear of aversive consequences, the approach may vary based on their inpatient or outpatient status. For those losing weight but not requiring hospitalization, it may be necessary to introduce a supplement immediately. Initial priorities for hospitalized patients and outpatients who can take a supplement should include exposing the patient to "newer-previously consumed items" and teaching and practicing productive coping strategies. Often a customized behavior modification plan is required to start to increase intake (see example in Chap. 10). As the patient progresses, the focus should shift toward building the routine of consuming adequate quantities, with consideration given to the Ladder Block Plan to reinforce intake. If the patient struggles with food quantity, priorities should include improving their ability to consume supplements, moving beyond their baseline food consumption (for example, setting goals to consume half an item if their baseline is only bites), and reintroducing eliminated items. The Ladder Block Plan should be considered if the patient is not consistently consuming enough quantity but meets the criteria for the plan, such as consuming at least 1000 kcal/day and taking at least 2 oz. of supplement at all meals and snacks.

Communicating Inpatient Feeding Plans for ARFID Patients

At our inpatient institution, occupational therapists (OTs) have developed and are responsible for creating a feeding plan tailored to each ARFID patient, providing a detailed and individualized approach to their care. The plan is bookmarked in the electronic medical record, allowing all team members to easily access it when needed. It includes a series of orders that differ from the standard AN-R treatment protocol. All of the above mentioned components, when relevant, are included in this plan. It is important that there is a system of clearly documenting the plan, as well as details of the patient's intake and eating behaviors, for all team members [9].

When possible, it's best for ARFID patients to work with core staff members who have experience and training with this population rather than staff who are floating from other units. See Chap. 22.

The goal of the feeding plan (see template Chap. 22) is to create an environment that supports the patient's success in increasing their nutritional intake. Like all OT plans, the aim is to develop the "just right challenge" [10] while progressively advancing the patient. For example, with patients with a fear of aversive consequences who are not at their baseline, it is often counterproductive to immediately implement an eat-replace plan. Typically, initially presenting food regularly and allowing the patient to choose how much to eat (i.e., ad lib plan) is more beneficial for these patients and for those with ARFID and sensory sensitivities. Conversely, for patients with ARFID-low interest, it may be advantageous to trial an eat-replace plan to assess their tolerance, as this approach can be easier to implement and, in some ways, less restrictive.

Order Sets That Support an Initial Feeding Plan

The below algorithm (Fig. 8.1) was created as a decision making tree for appropriate initial orders for patients based on their subtypes (as defined by the psych team); at our institution it is used on weekends when OT is not present. It could also be used as a tool at other institutions for choosing an initial plan for patients with different ARFID subtypes.

The Priority Conditions Nabla (Fig. 8.2) is a decision-making tool designed to help clinicians identify which conditions may most significantly influence a patient's behavior when more than one are present. It is an aid to the above algorithm. While it lists various conditions, the tool serves to aid in the selection of appropriate order sets based on observed symptoms and assessments. It does not replace clinical judgment.

How to use this tool: If the patient has more than one subtype noted by the diagnosing clinician, this Nabla can be used as a decision making aid to determine which orders are most appropriate. Choose the orders for the subtype closest to the top of the Nabla. For example, if both ARFID fear of aversive consequences and Anorexia Nervosa (AN) are present, the orders for ARFID fear of aversive consequences should be selected. If AN and ARFID-sensory are present, the standard orders for AN should be chosen.

Key Questions for Treatment Plan Development

Occupational therapists are required to develop treatment plans with goals that are measurable and time-bound. The following questions can help shape these treatment plans.

1. **How much inpatient time do you have with the patient?**

    - **3 days or less:** For patients with a limited stay, such as 3 days or less, it is crucial to maximize movement towards a safe feeding plan quickly. The occupational therapist (OT) should aim to taste-test a supplement on the same day

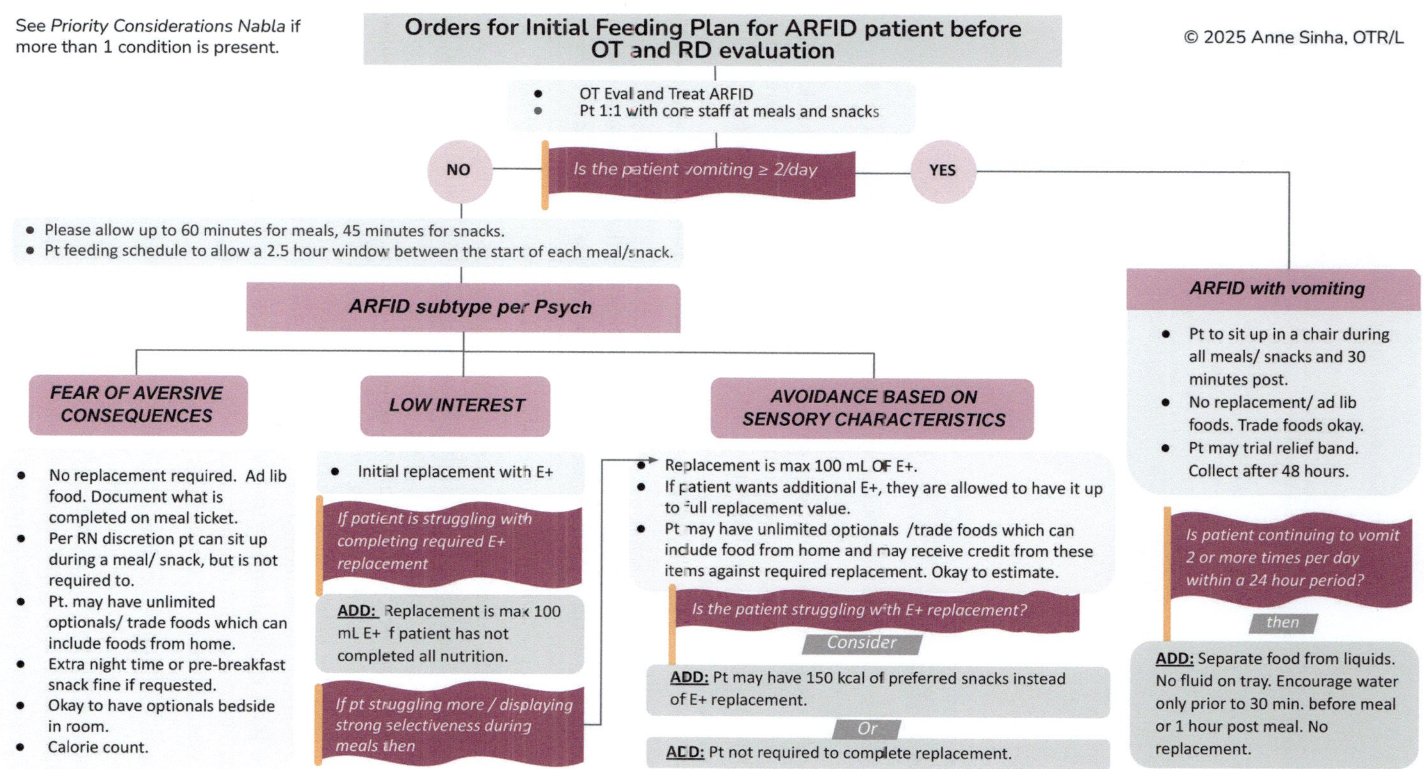

Fig. 8.1 Decision making tree for initial orders based on presented conditions

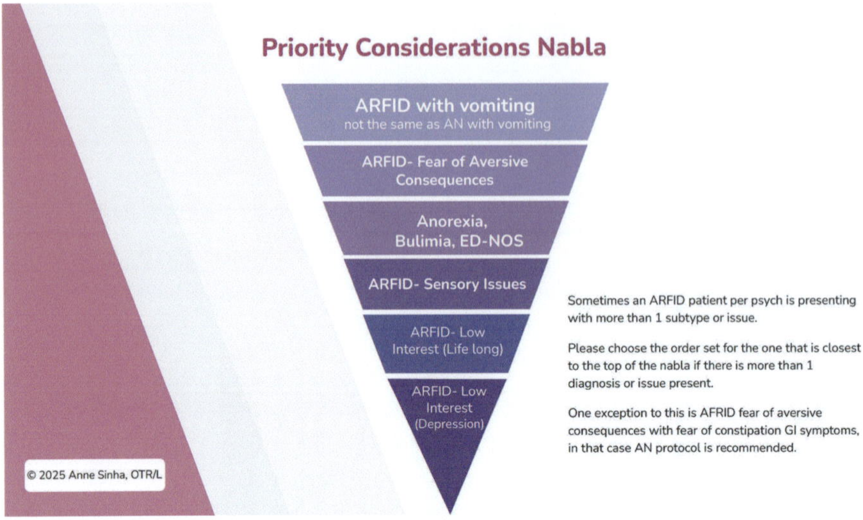

Fig. 8.2 The Priority Consideration Nabla is a tool to add the algorithm listed in Fig. 8.1

as the evaluation, ideally in a second feeding session (e.g., snack time) or during the first feeding session. For patients with sensory or low-interest ARFID, starting a supplement as early as possible can be valuable.

- **1 week:** If the patient has a week and exhibits fear issues, it may be beneficial to focus on food initially, as regaining food intake often requires more support than liquids.
- **2 weeks or more:** Longer durations allow for more flexibility and opportunities to observe the patient's baseline before starting a supplement.

2. **Are they in a position to tolerate a liquid (supplement) replacement?**

- **History with supplements:** Assess if the patient has had negative or positive experiences with supplements. For those with negative associations, and if the OT has at least 5 days, it is generally better to start with an ad lib plan of preferred foods for 24 h, also allowing for trade-ins of hospital shelf-available foods (e.g., graham crackers, yogurts, milk) and foods from home. Observe the patient's natural intake during this period.
- Taste testing supplements: On day 2 (or possibly day 1 if the stay is short), use the food exploration log to taste test different liquid supplements (1 ounce each is brought in) that are calorically equivalent to a 1.5 or higher.
- **Assess the patient's rankings:**

- Rank 3 or higher for "like it" section of the food exploration log: Identify the preferred supplement and consider an eat-replace model or 2 oz. at each meal and snack if they drank it easily.
- Difficulty drinking or consumed less than 1 ounce: Measure intake and, if less than 1 ounce, ask the patient if they can practice taking 15 mL at each meal and snack. If they took 1 ounce with difficulty, ask if they can repeat that at

each meal or snack. For those who took 1 ounce easily, discuss the eat-replace model versus 2 oz. at each meal and snack, and incorporate the patient's agreement into the bookmarked feeding plan.

- Once they tolerate a consistent supplement amount for 24 h, that can be increased, ideally step-by-step moving to a minimum of 2 ounces for 24 h in preparation for the Ladder Block Plan or an eat-replace model if the supplement becomes well tolerated.

A sample progression of a bookmarked feeding plan, applying the principles discussed above, can be found in the Chap. 22.

Through collaborative efforts, including meal observation, postural analysis, and oral motor skill assessment, occupational therapists can develop individualized feeding plans tailored to the unique needs of each ARFID patient. These tailored and adjustable plans address the specific challenges faced by each patient, promoting a gradual and sustainable improvement in nutritional intake. By fostering an environment conducive to patient progress, these strategies ensure that ARFID patients receive the comprehensive care necessary for long-term success.

The Ladder Block Plan

The Ladder Block Plan was created in 2018 by Anne Sinha, OTR/L, out of need for an ARFID patient who was not responding well to or understanding the value of the eat-replace model. This plan quickly demonstrated its utility for many subsequent ARFID patients. It is a novel paper-based behavior modification system designed to help ARFID patients overcome barriers to achieving full nutrition.

The plan features a unique visual reinforcement system that clearly segments nutritional needs and promotes a step-by-step process for meeting these needs. The behavior modification aspect occurs naturally, with or without additional rewards, due to its visual system. This system aligns well with the current trend of "gamification" and visualization, making it especially timely and useful for today's youth. Dietitians have found it beneficial, as it provides a level of clarity to both patients and their families, particularly for those with low interest in eating in cases where an eat-replace model has not been successful. Often, these patients or their families are unaware of the specific caloric requirements needed for the patient to thrive. The Ladder Block Plan addresses this by providing clear, visually reinforced information. Because of it's visual nature, team members can also see where a patient is falling behind and then may consider how to adjust the plan.

This behavior modification plan supports patients struggling with low weight to achieve adequate nourishment for health and wellness. The Ladder Block Plan is currently being developed into a broader digital IOS application for ARFID patients, called the Nourish Navigator. A beta version of this application will be tested at Stanford in 2026 .

The Ladder Block Plan

- Visual Behavior Modification Plan: The plan documents nutritional intake in a visually intuitive way.
- Blocks of the ladder: Each "block" represents a specific caloric amount
- Green Blocks: When nutritional blocks are met, the block is colored green.
- Yellow Blocks: If nutrition for a meal is missed and made up later, that portion of the block or blocks are colored yellow.
- Multiple Blocks: Some meals may require more than one nutritional block.
- Visual Reinforcers: Additional visual reinforcers are provided for obtaining all blocks and for getting all green blocks (indicating all nutrition was met at the planned time).
- Rewards for Younger Children: Block completion can result in points that can be used towards rewards (see Chap. 22 for a sample of a Ladder Block Plan with points).
- Blocks can be whole or ½ values: If a block is a ½ value, take the block value and divide it by 2. Block values do not go lower than ½.

Prior to starting the Ladder Block Plan:

- To begin the Ladder Block Plan, these criteria must be met first:
- Patient is having a minimum of 3 meals and 2 snack daily
- Patient is consuming 1000 + calories daily
- Patient is able to take 2 oz. of a supplement at each meal and snack for 24 hours (at times when the patients has issues with nausea or emesis the 2 oz. may not be offered at the breakfast or night snack interval. This would be planned in advance or in response to collected data and observations). See video for how to build this skill: Video 8.3.
- Parent is interested in using the plan and willing to support it's use

Video 8.3 Building the Skill of Taking a Supplement
https://youtu.be/ZNbO18jK6zY

For years, this plan was implemented visually without a written formula. Anne Sinha would assess the patient's caloric trends and divide the value of the blocks into increments ranging from 125–350 kcals providing 8–12 blocks/ day. The placement of the blocks was then determined by visually adjusting the distribution, ensuring that the overall caloric intake remained consistent or slightly increased from the previous day. This intuitive approach may work for some medical team members whereas others may develop this after using it for a while. However, if the intuitive approach does not work, until that proficiency is achieved, it is recommended to use the following formula:

1. **Establish a Baseline Intake**: Use either the average caloric intake from the past three days or the prior day's intake, whichever is higher. If using the 3-day average caloric intake, also calculate the average calories per meal and snack.
   * Eliminate anomalies of very high calorie meals (e.g., fast food meals) if not the norm. Instead take the typical calories consumed on prior days and add 100 kcals for the sample for that meal.
2. **Calculate the Block Quotient**: Take the Baseline Intake and divide it by 10, resulting in a quotient answer. (e.g., 2000/10 − 200 is the quotient).
3. **Assign Blocks to meals and Snacks**: Divide the calories of each individual meal and snack by the quotient:

   Example: Breakfast 423 kcal ÷ 200 = 2.12 blocks

4. **Round to the Nearest Block Value**:

   - < .74 → ½ block
   - 75–1.25 → 1 block
   - 1.26–1.74 → 1.5 blocks
   - 1.75–2.25 → 2 blocks
   - 2.26–2.74 → 2.5 blocks
   - 2.75–3.25 → 3 blocks
   - 3.26–3.74+ → 3.5 blocks

5. **Determine Number of Blocks**: Add total number of blocks.
6. **Determine Value of Each Block**: Cumulative caloric value of calories consumed rounded to the next 10 (i.e., 1 + equal to next 10, e.g., 1092 = 1110) + any calorie advancement (e.g., 100 kcals) / of blocks= caloric block value of each block (round to even number)
   Example: 1100+100=1200/ 10 = 120 kcal/ block
   A demonstration of how to apply this is found in (Table 8.1)

Table 8.1 Demonstration of how to apply the ladder block plan formula using a sample scenario with a resulting ladder block plan (Fig. 8.3)

Meals	Day 1	Day 2	Day3	3-day Average	Meal Kcals/ Quotient	Resulting answer to determine # of blocks	Blocks/meal per formula	Resulting calories/ blocks and total if keeping values the same	Resulting calories/ block if advancing calories by 100 kcals that day
Caloric value/ block								1100/10 = 110 kcal/block	1200/10 = 120 kcal/block
Breakfast kcals	200	220	210	210	210/110	1.9	2 blocks	2 blocks = 220 kcals	2 blocks = 240 kcals
Lunch kcals	350	331	345	342	342/110	3.1	3 blocks	3 blocks = 330 kcals	3 blocks = 360 kcals
Afternoon Snack kcals	100	101	110	104	104/110	.94	1 block	1 block = 110 kcals	1 block = 120 kcals
Dinner kcals	300	350	336	329	329/110	2.99	3 blocks	3 blocks = 330 kcal	3 blocks = 360 kcal
Night snack kcals	100	120	100	107	107/110	.97	1 block	1 block = 110 kcals	1 block = 120 kcals
Cumulative value	1050	1122	1101	1092			10 blocks	1100 kcal 10 locks	1200 kcal 10 blocks

Day:	Day:	Day:	Day:	Day:	Day:	Day:
Used Strategies	Used Strategies	Used Strategies	Used Strategies	Used Strategies	Used Strategies	Used Strategies
All green	All green	All green	All green	All green	All green	All green
All met	All met	All met	All met	All met	All met	All met
Night snack	Night snack	Night snack	Night snack	Night snack	Night snack	Night snack
Dinner	Dinner	Dinner	Dinner	Dinner	Dinner	Dinner
Dinner	Dinner	Dinner	Dinner	Dinner	Dinner	Dinner
Dinner	Dinner	Dinner	Dinner	Dinner	Dinner	Dinner
Afternoon Snack	Afternoon Snack	Afternoon Snack	Afternoon Snack	Afternoon Snack	Afternoon Snack	Afternoon Snack
Lunch	Lunch	Lunch	Lunch	Lunch	Lunch	Lunch
Lunch	Lunch	Lunch	Lunch	Lunch	Lunch	Lunch
Lunch	Lunch	Lunch	Lunch	Lunch	Lunch	Lunch
Breakfast	Breakfast	Breakfast	Breakfast	Breakfast	Breakfast	Breakfast
Breakfast	Breakfast	Breakfast	Breakfast	Breakfast	Breakfast	Breakfast
Extra kcals:	Extra kcals:	Extra kcals:	Extra kcals:	Extra kcals:	Extra kcals:	Extra kcals:

Fig. 8.3 Ladder block plan derived from the sample scenario in Table 8.1

Ladder Block Plan

Sheet to track meeting nutritional needs to support brain and body optimal function

Friday	Saturday	Sunday	Monday	Tuesday	Wednesday	Thursday
Used strategies	Used strategies	Used strategies	Used strategies	Used strategies	Used strategies	Used strategies
All green	All green	All green	All green	All green	All green	All green
All met	All met	All met	All met	All met	All met	All met
Snack	Snack	Snack	Snack	Snack	Snack	Snack
Dinner 1/2	Dinner 1/2	Dinner 1/2	Dinner 1/2	Dinner 1/2	Dinner 1/2	Dinner 1/2
Dinner	Dinner	Dinner	Dinner	Dinner	Dinner	Dinner
Dinner	Dinner	Dinner	Dinner	Dinner	Dinner	Dinner
Snack	Snack	Snack	Snack	Snack	Snack	Snack
Lunch 1/2	Lunch 1/2	Lunch 1/2	Lunch 1/2	Lunch 1/2	Lunch 1/2	Lunch 1/2
Lunch	Lunch	Lunch	Lunch	Lunch	Lunch	Lunch
Lunch	Lunch	Lunch	Lunch	Lunch	Lunch	Lunch
Breakfast1/2	Breakfast1/2	Breakfast1/2	Breakfast1/2	Breakfast1/2	Breakfast1/2	Breakfast 1/2
Breakfast	Breakfast	Breakfast	Breakfast	Breakfast	Breakfast	Breakfast
Extra kcals:	Extra kcals:	Extra kcals:	Extra kcals:	Extra kcals:	Extra kcals:	Extra kcals:

Ladder Block Instructions

- Each meal/ snack block represents "a block of nutrition" per RD guidelines of specific caloric value/ block.
- Please color block Green when completed at meal, Yellow when completed at a later meal.
- Please note that coloring the full amount in green represents getting all required nutrition at that mealtime with any nutritional source.
- Food items may be exchanged or replaced with other food items or supplement (if desired).
- It is important to keep rotating food items to avoid food jags.
- If more kcals are achieved during a meal than the block needs, record the extra value in the bottom "extra kcal" section, they may be used to complete later blocks as needed/desired (within the same day only).
- Only color in complete block(s) if that full nutritional value is consumed at that meal or used in combination with the "extra kcal" calories. When those are used, cross them off to indicate they have been utilized.
- If blocks are not fully completed at any meal, color only up to what has been completed, leaving that section blank, if made up later (by going over at a subsequent meal or snack and giving caloric credit), color in yellow.
- Always first color the blocks for that meal/ snack before making up nutrition from a prior meal.

Why Is It Called "The Ladder Block Plan? And Why Does It Move from the Bottom Up?"

Just like you climb a ladder from the bottom to the top, that is how you move with the Ladder Block Plan. The bottom represents the start of the day. The rungs are symbolized by the lines that build the bottom and top of the blocks. As you achieve "each block" of nutrition, you "climb the rungs of the ladder" as you meet your nutritional needs for the day. The goal is to climb each rung, achieving all nutrition by coloring in the blocks green, as you reach the top! This symbolizes meeting your full nutritional needs on that day.

Considerations About the Ladder Block Plan

Even if the patient tends toward consuming a significant amount of nutrition during nighttime snacks, it may be beneficial to slightly understate the nighttime blocks to allow for the potential to "make up blocks" later with the nighttime nutrition. If a patient starts advancing their nutrition by consistently eating more at a certain time of day, it may be necessary to reconfigure the blocks accordingly to reflect patient trends.

Fig. 8.4 Partial Sample of a Flexible Block Plan Combining Lunch and Snack

Snack	Snack
Afternoon Snack	Afternoon Snack
Lunch/Snack 1/2	Lunch/Snack 1/2
Lunch/Snack	Lunch/Snack
Lunch	Lunch

Particularly during hospitalization, when determining what the patient will eat, it can be helpful to send more nutrition than what would be needed to "just make the block." This approach gives the patient an opportunity to find foods they like and to exceed the block value if the food is enjoyed, which can enable the meal plan to be advanced more quickly.

There are times when an ARFID patient starts struggling with advancing their breakfast nutrition (or nutrition for another time of day). When this occurs, modifications may need to be made by reducing blocks at that time and adding blocks elsewhere. Sometimes the block plan needs to be different for school days versus non-school days or when custody is shared between two parents, based on the trends for that household. Blocks can sometimes be indicated as Lunch/Snack or Snack/Dinner to allow more flexibility in these situations, or the block plan can vary by day or situation. For example, some school children's consumption at school lunch may be more like a snack and a full meal upon getting home, whereas on weekends they eat a full meal at lunch and then an afternoon snack. The plan could show flexibility as listed below (Fig. 8.4).

If not using the formula and configuring mentally, it is important when the patient is on a low caloric level (e.g., 1000–1500 calories) to make the initial block value low so there is space to advance as the patient advances their meal plan.

At times, the block placement may have a different configuration. For example, for college students who stay up late and sleep late, their blocks may start with lunch, and they may have two dinner-type meals in the night. The plan should be adapted to the patient's unique needs and trends to support their success. If this approach does not work, then the patient may need education about the value of shifting their schedule back so nutrition can start earlier in the day.

Advancing Individual Block Value to Increase Total Calories

If the Patient Is Quickly Advancing Their Nutrition

While inpatient and increasing total caloric intake, it is recommended to graph the calories consumed at each meal and snack, as shown in sample Table 8.2. This helps track whether the patient is consistently making progress at individual meals and throughout the day. At our institution, the RN includes a note in the electronic

Table 8.2 Sample of graph showing calories consumed at each meal and snack

	Monday	Tuesday	Wednesday
Breakfast kcals	393	280	413
Lunch kcals	438	695	801
Afternoon snack kcals	375	345	382
Dinner kcals	328	310	381
Night snack kcals	360	398	476
Cumulative kcal value	1894	2028	2453

medical record system (per the bookmarked feeding plan) that states the caloric value at each meal and snack; this information is used to graph calories.

When the patient consistently achieves all green blocks (meeting all nutritional goals), tolerates the increase well, and the RD supports advancement, the individual block value can be increased to raise the total caloric intake. For example, if a patient consumes a total of 2230 calories, this can be rounded up to 2300 calories for ease of calculation. The new individual block value is then calculated by dividing the total calories by the number of blocks (e.g., 2300 calories divided by 10 blocks equals 230 calories per block).

If the Patient Is not Meeting Their Blocks or Struggling
If the patient fails to meet their block goals or experiences nausea or pain, it is recommended to maintain the current block value (or occasionally reduce the block value) for 24 h and provide additional support through productive coping strategies and problem-solving.

If the Patient Is Achieving but not Exceeding Their Blocks
If the patient is "just making" their blocks, it is acceptable to advance up to 100 kcals if the patient feels ready and supports the increase. Though 200 kcal/day advancements are common for AN-R patients, for ARFID patients, the average is 100 kcal/day unless the patient advances themselves more quickly.

Outpatient Considerations
While in outpatient care, it is more common to advance every 2–7 days when the patient is meeting or exceeding their nutritional goals. Parents (or the patient) can be taught to support advancing the plan by monitoring trends and increasing the block value by 10 calories per block when the patient is ready.

Developing a feeding plan for the patient and family supports their progress by setting clear expectations and guidelines. Parents have an important role in the feeding plan by establishing regular meals and snacks and supporting the patient in their use of productive coping strategies. Communication with the broader team is important to ensure the feeding plan is effective. Reinforcing the feeding plan through the Ladder Block Plan or other behavior modification strategies can accelerate the patient's progress and support their success.

References

1. Lawrence SD, Plisco MK. Family mealtimes and family functioning. Am J Fam Ther. 2017;45(4):1–11. https://doi.org/10.1080/01926187.2017.1328991.
2. Middleton G, Golley RK, Patterson KA, Coveney J. The family meal framework: a grounded theory study conceptualizing the work that underpins the family meal. Appetite. 2022;175:106071. https://doi-org.laneproxy.stanford.edu/10.1016/j.appet.2022.106071
3. Cosbey J, Muldoon D. EAT-UP™ family-centered feeding intervention to promote food acceptance and decrease challenging behaviors: a single-case experimental design replicated across three families of children with autism spectrum disorder. J Autism Dev Disord. 2017;47(3):564–78. https://doi-org.laneproxy.stanford.edu/10.1007/s10803-016-2977-0
4. Gray JM. Putting occupation into practice: occupation as ends, occupation as means. Am J Occup Ther. 1998;52(5):354–64. https://doi-org.laneproxy.stanford.edu/10.5014/ajot.52.5.354
5. Pyatak EA, Carandang K, Rice Collins C, Carlson M. Optimizing occupations, habits, and routines for health and well-being with Lifestyle Redesign®: a synthesis and scoping review. Am J Occup Ther. 2022;76(5):7605205050. https://doi.org/10.5014/ajot.2022.049269.
6. Yoshikawa M, Nagakawa K, Tanaka R, Yamawaki K, Mori T, Hiraoka A, Higa C, Nishikawa Y, Yoshida M, Tsuga K. Improper sitting posture while eating adversely affects maximum tongue pressure. J Dent Sci. 2021;16(1):467–73. https://doi-org.laneproxy.stanford.edu/10.1016/j.jds.2020.08.012
7. American Occupational Therapy Association. Specialized knowledge and skills in feeding, eating, and swallowing for occupational therapy practice. Am J Occup Ther. 2007;61(6):686–700. https://doi.org/10.5014/ajot.61.6.686.
8. Kielhofner G. Temporal adaptation: a conceptual framework for occupational therapy. Am J Occup Ther. 1977;31(4):235–42.
9. Gorrell S, Vendlinski SS, Thompson AS, Downey AE, Kramer R, Hail L, Clifton S, Forsberg S, Reilly EE, Saunders E, Buckelew SM, Le Grange D. Modification of an inpatient medical management protocol for pediatric avoidant/restrictive food intake disorder: improving the standard of care. J Eat Disord. 2023;11(1):165. https://doi-org.laneproxy.stanford.edu/10.1186/s40337-023-00895-9
10. Kuhaneck H, Spitzer SL. The importance of conceptual origins: the case of the just-right challenge. Am J Occup Ther. 2024;78(4):7804185110. https://doi-org.laneproxy.stanford.edu/10.5014/ajot.2024.050619

Chapter 9
Behavioral Modification

Behavior Modification Plans

Behavior modification is a valuable tool for helping ARFID patients [1] and their families develop the skills needed to ensure the patient consistently receives adequate nutrition. It reinforces behaviors that align with treatment goals [2] and builds on informal behavior management strategies that parents already employ, such as requiring children to complete their homework before playing video games. By developing a more structured behavior modification plan, these existing practices are expanded to support the patient in achieving consistent nutrition and broader treatment objectives.

Before implementing a formal behavior modification plan, it is important to discuss its purpose and potential rewards with the parents [3]. Positive reinforcement is recommended, and therapists should collaborate closely with families to ensure that the chosen methods align with treatment goals and effectively support the patient's progress.

To introduce a plan, one might say to the parent, "Based on our observations, a behavior modification plan could accelerate your child's progress.Such a plan outlines specific meal and snack goals, with a reward component to motivate and track progress. Is this something you're open to discussing?"

If the parent agrees, further details on the theory of behavioral modification and suitable rewards are discussed. It's important that rewards are meaningful, reasonable and affordable, controllable by parents, and not already accessible to the child (e.g., additional screen time beyond baseline usage). In cases of significant progress, adjustments may be considered. There are times when parents like the idea of a chart to track progress but prefer not to attach rewards.

A. Sinha et al., *Comprehensive Clinical Care for Adolescents with Avoidant/Restrictive Food Intake Disorder (ARFID)*,
https://doi.org/10.1007/978-3-031-92232-9_9

Key Components of a Behavior Modification Plan

Parental Commitment: Confirm that parents are willing and capable of consistently executing the plan.

Realistic Goal Setting: Conduct initial feeding sessions to assess current eating patterns and agree on achievable goals.

Immediate and Controlled Rewards: Ensure rewards are readily administered by parents and effectively motivate the child.

Examples of Rewards

- **Money:** Money can be an effective motivator for many patients [4]. Discuss with parents how much the child can earn per week. Parents need to feel empowered to choose an amount that they can afford and make sure this aligns with their values as a family. Typically, moderate amounts between $7 and $20 per week are adequate to be motivating, without being excessive. Adjustments can be made if the patient shows significant or unexpected progress. Deciding where and when the money can be spent on a specific reward can be an added motivation.
- **Controlled Screen Time or Games**: Screen time or games on a parent-controlled device (e.g., a parent's iPhone) can be effective. The parent should have complete control over access and duration, ensuring the reward is time-bound and not readily accessible to the patient.
- **Reward Events with Parents**: Special events are suitable only if parents can consistently allocate time for these activities. These should be additional events that do not occur regularly. At times these can be more challenging to provide consistently compared to financial rewards.
- **Special Choices:** Earning the right to choose the evening's media, select a game to play, pick a park to visit, or decide on an outing.
- **Bonus Playdates:** Some youth may be motivated to earn extra opportunities to have friends come over that go beyond typical opportunities.
- **Occasional Special Foods**: Special foods that are not typically available can sometimes be effective rewards, even for patients that are working on increasing nutrition.
- **Game Money**: Virtual currency added to a video game portal can be motivating for patients who value gaming.
- **Gift Certificates**: Certificates for specific stores or online platforms allow the patient to select their rewards within defined limits.
- **Toys or Treats for Pets**: Items for a family pet that are not usually given can serve as unique rewards.
- **Hospital Gift Shop Visits**: In a hospital setting, a daily trip to the gift shop can be motivating as it allows the patient to see something new and may help them plan for an item they are motivated to earn.
- **Collectible Cards**: Pokémon cards or similar collectibles can be effective, especially for patients with a strong interest in such items.

- **Picture Printouts**: Printouts of favorite artists, scenes, or characters can also be motivating rewards.
- **Prize Bag Prizes**: Items from a prize bag or prizes with assigned point values can work well, depending on the patient's interests.

Inappropriate Rewards

Certain rewards should be avoided due to their impracticality or potential to undermine the behavior modification plan:

- **Large Rewards**: Rewards such as earning a pet or a major trip (e.g., to Disney) can be unrealistic and may detract from the effectiveness of the behavior modification plan.
- **Baseline Expectations**: Avoid rewards that take away something already part of the patient's routine, such as general time with a parent or screen time that is already granted.
- **Allowances**: Additional money earned through the behavior modification plan should be separate from the child's regular allowance and not alter the baseline amount.

Behavior modification plans should be based on observed eating behaviors during sessions. It is important to set achievable goals that help patients to step-by-step move beyond their baseline to encourage patient progress without overwhelming them. Often it can be useful to bring a reward plan to one meal only before creating the chart for the subsequent twenty-four or more hour period. This can allow the therapist and parent to determine if the plan appears viable.

Once the therapist has observed the patient during a meal, they can develop a behavior modification plan based on the patient's presentation. When prioritizing behavioral expectations, the top priority for outpatients who are losing weight is reinforcing regular nutrition intake from any source to avoid further weight loss and potential hospitalization.

The ARFID subtype and the setting (inpatient versus outpatient) can significantly impact the priorities of the behavior modification plan. For every subtype, reinforcing the use of productive coping strategies is a priority.

Important Components of Using a Behavior Modification Plan

1. Fill out the plan after every eating interval.
2. Add up the points at the end of each day
3. Make sure rewards are provided as soon as they are earned

Considering the priorities for each patient, which can be influenced with knowledge of their ARFID subtype can help when designing behavior modification plans. Please note that this is a general guide based on trends. Individual presentation of the patient while eating with them is the best way to determine just right challenges for a behavior modification plan.

Outpatient and Inpatient-ARFID Low Interest Behavior Modification

- Prioritize creating a regular schedule of eating.
- Starting a supplement, if taken easily move to eat-replace protocol.
- Reinforce quantity.
- Trial natural rewards and scheduling (e.g., let's eat before going to the park or having screen time) before a formal behavior modification system. See Fig. 9.1 for sample behavior modification plan.

Example 1

Below (Fig. 9.1) is a sample behavior modification chart designed to initially reinforce food quantity, supplement intake and the use of strategies in a patient who struggles with food quantity but not variety (e.g., low interest). Note that the quantity of the supplement is not defined in a behavior modification plan in case it increases; however, patients are informed if there is a set amount that increases. If the supplement is intended to relace missed nutrition, the goal would instead state "took replacement." Initially, 1 ounce of a supplement was provided when the patient did not finish her food (which was 100% of the time). Gradually, it increases to 2 oz. and eventually this goal was changed to taking replacement (of whatever nutrition she needed to meet the nutritional goal of that meal set by the dietitian).

Outpatient ARFID Sensory Behavior Modification

- Use Food Exploration Log to reinforce return of previously eaten foods and newer foods with option of reward component (see Chap 22; Appendix N).
- Parents may also keep a log of having presented "1 new" and 2–4 familiar items at snacks, meals. This helps parents become accountable and build a new skill of presenting other foods.
- Start with small quantities of a supplement and build up with reward component.

Inpatient ARFID Sensory Behavior Modification

- Behavior modification to reinforce quality and starting a supplement and "tried a newer food," see sample Chart. 9.1.

Outpatient ARFID-Fear of Aversive Consequences Behavior Modification

- If losing weight but not requiring hospitalization, consider using a supplement immediately and provide points for it's completion.
- Start of food exposure/handling. The Food Exploration Log can be helpful with or without points (Chap 7, Chap 22 Appendix N).
- Ensure adequate quantity, consider ladder block plan to reinforce quantity.

Inpatient ARFID-Fear of Aversive Consequences Behavior Modification

- Food exposure to "newer-previously consumed items "(i.e., food the patient liked and ate regularly prior to their fear)."
- Use of productive coping strategies.
- Priorities for Progressing Nutrition (If Struggling with Food Quantity).
- Ability to take a supplement.
- Moving beyond their baseline in food consumption (e.g., may set goals of consuming a ½ item if baseline is bites).
- Regaining eliminated items.
- Consider ladder block plan if not consistently getting enough quantity but meeting the criteria for the plan (i.e., 1000 + kcals/ day and 2 oz. + supplement at all meals and snacks).

	Day:	Day:
Breakfast 1 point each	Completed 25% of nutrition: Completed 50% of nutrition: Completed 75% of nutrition: Completed all nutrition: Took provided supplement: Used strategies:	Completed 25% of nutrition: Completed 50% of nutrition: Completed 75% of nutrition: Completed all nutrition: Took provided supplement: Used strategies:
Lunch 1 point each	Completed 25% of nutrition: Completed 50% of nutrition: Completed 75% of nutrition: Completed all nutrition: Took provided supplement:	Completed 25% of nutrition: Completed 50% of nutrition: Completed 75% of nutrition: Completed all nutrition: Took provided supplement:
	Used strategies:	Used strategies:
Afternoon Snack 1 point each	Completed 25% of nutrition: Completed 50% of nutrition: Completed 75% of nutrition: Completed all nutrition: Took provided supplement: Used strategies:	Completed 25% of nutrition: Completed 50% of nutrition: Completed 75% of nutrition: Completed all nutrition: Took provided supplement: Used strategies:
Dinner 1 point each	Completed 25% of nutrition: Completed 50% of nutrition: Completed 75% of nutrition: Completed all nutrition: Took provided supplement: Used strategies:	Completed 25% of nutrition: Completed 50% of nutrition: Completed 75% of nutrition: Completed all nutrition: Took provided supplement: Used strategies:
Night snack 1 point each	Completed 25% of nutrition: Completed 50% of nutrition: Completed 75% of nutrition: Completed all nutrition: Took provided supplement: Used strategies:	Completed 25% of nutrition: Completed 50% of nutrition: Completed 75% of nutrition: Completed all nutrition: Took provided supplement: Used strategies:
Total Earned		
Total Used		
Total Remaining		

Fig. 9.1 Behavior modification chart that reinforces quantity, supplement completion and the use of productive coping strategies

Breakfast	Completed ½ item (1 pt/ each): Completed full item (1 pt/ each): Took supplement (1 pt): 3+ bites of a newer food (1 pt/ item): Used strategies (1 pt):
Lunch	Completed ½ item (1 pt/ each): Took supplement (1 pt): 3+ bites of a newer food (1 pt/ item): Used strategies (1 pt):
Snack	Completed ½ item (1 pt/ each): Took supplement (1 pt): 3+ bites of a newer food (1 pt/ item): Used strategies (1 pt):
Dinner	Completed ½ item (1 pt/ each): Took supplement (1 pt): 3+ bites of a newer food (1 pt/ item): Used strategies (1 pt):
Snack	Completed ½ item (1 pt/ each): Took supplement (1 pt): 3+ bites of a newer food (1 pt/ item): Used strategies (1 pt):
Today's total points	
Yesterday's points	
Points used	
Cumulative points	

Interpreting points: Completed ½ item= ½ item of any food per parent/ RN discretion

Completed full item (1 pt/ each): 1 pt for complete item finished, can get ½ and full point

Took supplement: Completed 100% of provided supplement (see medical order for quantity)

3+ bites of newer food (1 pt/ item): 3+ bites (any size) of newer foods refer to foods trialed in the hospital for the first 5+ times (different brands, types) or foods pt has not had for 1+ month. Use Food Exploration Log

Used strategies (1 pt/ feeding session): Pt uses any 1+ defined strategies on their coping strategies list: e.g., Start with a bite, use of change-taste food, straw breath, see list for more

Reward: 25 pt = $1 to spend at gift shop or on Amazon

Chart. 9.1 Behavior Modification Chart that reinforces increasing quantity through bites, items, supplement completion and use of strategies

Example 2

Below (Fig. 9.2) is a portion of an initial behavior modification plan (for brevity, not all meals are included, but they were part of the actual chart) for an ARFID fear of aversive consequences patient experiencing acute food refusal. At the time this plan was created, the patient could barely sit in front of a tray:

This (Fig. 9.3) was a portion of the second behavior modification chart for the patient with acute food refusal.

The patient's behavior modification chart was advanced (Fig. 9.4) as the patient progressed.

Figure 9.5 shows the next chart that was used as the patient progressed.

Figure 9.6 shows the next chart that was used as the patient progressed.

Figure 9.7 shows the next chart that was used as the patient progressed.

	Day:	Day:	Day:
	Complete breathing technique practice (1 pt/ each):	Complete breathing technique practice (1 pt/ each):	Complete breathing technique practice (1 pt/ each):
Meal:	Lift up food (1 pt)= Touch food to mouth (1 pt)= Lick food item (2 pt)= Bite(s) of food (5 pt/item)= Used strategies (1 pt)=	Lift up food (1 pt)= Touch food to mouth (1 pt)= Lick food item (2 pt)= Bite(s) of food (5 pt/item)= Used strategies (1 pt)=	Lift up food (1 pt)= Touch food to mouth (1 pt)= Lick food item (2 pt)= Bite(s) of food (5 pt/item)= Used strategies (1 pt)=

Fig. 9.2 Initial behavior modification for patient in acute food refusal

	Day:	Day:
	Drank provided water (2 pt):	Drank provided water (2 pt):
Meal:	Brought food to own lips (1 pt)= Lick food item (1 pt)= Bite(s)/swallow food (2 pt/ item)= Used strategies (1 pt)=	Brought food to own lips (1 pt)= Lick food item (1 pt)= Bite(s)/swallow food (2 pt/ item)= Used strategies (1 pt)=

Fig. 9.3 Behavior modification plan 2 progressed for patient in acute food refusal

	Day:
	Drank provided water (2 pt):
MEAL	Lick food item (1 pt)= Bite(s)/swallow food (1 pt/ item)= Eat small food item (2pt)= Used strategies (1 pt)=

Fig. 9.4 Behavior modification plan 3 progressed for patient in acute food refusal

	DAY:
	Drank provided water (2 pt)=
	Drank provided juice/milk (2 pt)=
Meal	Lick NEW food item (1 pt)= Eat spoonful of food (1 pt)= Eat 2 small food items (1 pt)= Eat ¼ main food (2 pts)= Used strategies (1 pt)=

Fig. 9.5 Behavior modification plan 4 progressed for patient in acute food refusal

	Day:
Completed water bottle (5)	
	Drank provided juice/milk (2 pt)=
Meal	Lick NEW food item (1 pt)= 3 bites new item (1 pt)= Eat ¼ food portion (1 pts)= Completed food item (5 pt/item)= Used strategies (1 pt)=

Fig. 9.6 Behavior modification plan 5 progressed for patient in acute food refusal

	Day:
Pill swallowing practice (1 pt/ practice time)	
Completed water bottle (5 pt)	
	Drank provided juice/milk (2 pt)=
Meal	3 bites new item (1 pt)= Eat 1/2 food portion (1 pts)= Completed food item (5 pt/item)= Used strategies (1 pt)= Complete supplement (1 pt)=

Fig. 9.7 Behavior modification plan 6 progressed for patient in acute food refusal

NEXT STEP

Once the patient had achieved 1000 + calories per day and was able to take 2 ounces of a supplement at each meal and snack, they were then moved to a Ladder Block Plan and their intake gradually progressed (see Chap. 8 for Ladder Block Plan use).

Behavior modification, when tailored to the patient's needs and implemented collaboratively with parents, can significantly enhance eating behaviors in ARFID patients. By focusing on achievable goals and meaningful rewards, therapists can support consistent progress and positive outcomes.

References

1. McMahon MXH, Hathaway KL, Hodges AK, Sharp WG, Volkert VM. A retrospective consecutive controlled case series of underspoon: a modified-bolus placement to address behavior that interfere with swallowing. Behavior Modification. 2023;47(4):870–904. https://doi-org.laneproxy.stanford.edu/10.1177/01454455221129996
2. Miltenberger RG. Behavior modification: principles and procedures. 6th ed. Cengage Learning; 2016.
3. Matthys W, Schutter DJLG. Involving parents in cognitive behavioral therapy for children and adolescents with conduct problems: goals, outcome expectations, and normative beliefs about aggression are targeted in sessions with parents and their child. Clinical Child Family Psychol Rev. 2024;27(2):561–75. https://doi-org.laneproxy.stanford.edu/10.1007/s10567-024-00486-3
4. Li HX, Long QS, Chen AT, Li Q. Sheng li xue bao: [Acta physiologica Sinica]. 2019;71(4):562–74. https://pubmed-ncbi-nlm-nih-gov.laneproxy.stanford.edu/31440753/

Chapter 10
Building a Multidisciplinary Team

ARFID: Importance of a Multidisciplinary Team

When managing patients with ARFID, as for many complex diagnoses, having a multidisciplinary team is critical. Depending on the resources available to you and the specific needs of the patient, the team's composition and team members' disciplines may look slightly different. When resources are lacking, a team member of one specialty may need to play the role of another. However, it is always ideal to identify a team who can work together and bring their expertise to optimize patient care.

Depending on the clinical needs of the patient, certain services may play more of a primary role as opposed to a supporting one. While in person visits may be preferred by some families, resources may not always be available. Fortunately, many providers are able to do virtual visits which can enable a team to be larger than what might be supported by geographic location. This can also provide the opportunity for the patient to work with a more experienced team.

Examples of team members to consider when managing a patient with ARFID:

Medical clinician: Often the first point of contact for patients and families, the clinician's role is to ensure that the appropriate primary diagnoses have been made and other potential diagnoses have been ruled out. In addition, the clinician is assessing for medical complications related to malnutrition that might require specific interventions. While not always necessary, it can be helpful to consult with an eating disorder specialist for assessment and ongoing management recommendations.

Mental health clinician: ARFID is a psychiatric diagnosis, so these clinicians are responsible for the diagnostic assessment of the eating disorder and co-occurring conditions such as anxiety or depression, which may result in additional challenges to managing the underlying ARFID disorder. For those patients who may benefit from psychotropic medication, having a psychiatric prescriber who is knowledgeable about ARFID and comorbid conditions is critical. A psychotherapist with expertise in ARFID treatment is an important part of the treatment team. Sometimes, a psychiatrist will act in both capacities.

A. B. Sinha et al., *Comprehensive Clinical Care for Adolescents with Avoidant/Restrictive Food Intake Disorder (ARFID)*,
https://doi.org/10.1007/978-3-031-92232-9_10

Dietitian: Working with a dietitian skilled in managing the nutritional needs of growing children and adolescents is important for setting appropriate nutritional goals and recommendations. Not all dietitians are familiar with working with ARFID patients and the needs that vary based on ARFID-subtype, so it is important to identify providers with this expertise.

Occupational Therapist: An occupational therapist who is knowledgeable in specifics for managing ARFID patients is enormously helpful. Depending on the region and availability of resources in the community, in addition or alternatively a Speech therapist may also assist with treating ARFID patients.

When managing a patient in the inpatient setting, having a daily huddle or rounds where all team members can connect and collaborate on a care plan is very helpful. Identifying each member's role (such as who is directing the calorie level or managing the behavior plan), as well as providing opportunities to discuss when plans are not working and need to be adapted, can manage team dynamics in a helpful manner. In the ambulatory setting, it is unusual for team members to have immediate access to each other. However, identifying members and having opportunities to connect between visits (such as utilizing secure messaging groups) can enable management plans to progress.

If needing to identify providers to build a team for management of patients with ARFID, there are several means to assess resources that may be available locally or virtually. For local therapists with eating disorder experience, consider searching the website Psychology Today for appropriate individuals. Academic centers with adolescent medicine divisions and/or psychiatry departments can be excellent sources of referral information. Local eating disorder resource centers or coalitions, as well as the Academy for Eating Disorders, have on-line resources for provider searches, as well.

Finally, talking with other families who have navigated the ARFID landscape of providers can often provide insightful suggestions.

Chapter 11
Insurance Coverage

While the ARFID diagnosis is new to the DSM-5, patients meeting criteria for ARFID have always existed. Many of them were treated in gastroenterology clinics and diagnosed as having failure to thrive or a specific food related phobia.

As clinicians become more familiar with the ARFID diagnosis, it is becoming easier to find providers with experience treating the disorder. Eating disorders specialists are more routinely exposed to ARFID patients during their training, and programs offering higher levels of care increasingly have focused ARFID tracks. Most of these programs have in network contracts with commercial insurance companies, and many are willing to create single case agreements with government payors.

That being said, some patients have had chronic symptoms over many years that have not been properly treated. Many parents were told that their child would grow out of their symptoms, only to see them become more entrenched over time. Weekly psychotherapy visits or even intensive partial hospital or residential programming with clinicians experienced in ARFID may not be available in their community. If available, programs may not be adequate for the severity of symptoms or specific needs of a particular patient.

Inpatient medical stabilization and psychiatric units specializing in eating disorders may be necessary to provide the support and structure needed to help an individual make meaningful progress in treatment. Sometimes, hospitalization helps families develop a sense of urgency about the need to make change as well as providing immersion in highly structured meals and snacks with behavioral interventions to help them really internalize and cement the changes necessary. However, units with significant ARFID expertise are rare, and there is variability in their approach.

Inpatient psychiatric hospitalization will likely require a pre-authorization with the behavioral health carve out of the insurance company to make sure that the patient requires inpatient level of care. When a patient is medically unstable (see

A. B. Sinha et al., *Comprehensive Clinical Care for Adolescents with Avoidant/Restrictive Food Intake Disorder (ARFID)*,
https://doi.org/10.1007/978-3-031-92232-9_11

Chap. 4), an inpatient medical admission is warranted and typically covered by insurance due to the acute medical instability. Unfortunately, the patient will need to discharge when they stabilize. This may give families a very limited time in the hospital to take advantage of the milieu and customized programming. If a patient is medically stable, it can be more challenging to obtain insurance coverage for higher levels of care.

In order to give the team adequate time to complete a comprehensive assessment and develop a customized plan to target the specific ARFID subtype and co-occurring conditions, a pre-authorization for a meaningful inpatient stay is often necessary. A referring primary care or specialty provider may be able to initiate a pre-authorization request with the insurance company to request adequate time to make progress with the needed treatment. Medical social workers and/or case managers should be able to assist with the process, and it helps when parents are able to pull together summaries describing treatment accessed thus far. It is important to build a narrative in support of the level of care being requested. Why is this level of care necessary?

1. Determine the type of hospitalization being requested. If the unit is an inpatient medical unit (as opposed to some eating disorder units which are psychiatric hospitals), the request will need to be initiated with the medical insurance and NOT with the behavioral health carve out.
2. Gather clinical information to build the case about the need for hospitalization. Why does the individual require an inpatient level of structure and support?
    (a) How long have the eating issues been present?
    (b) What is the patient/family understanding of the illness and what is their motivation for change?
    (c) Has the family participated in previous eating disorder treatment in the past?
        (i) What types of programming (it helps to have program names, level of care and dates of treatment)?
        (ii) Were treatment attempts adequate and did patient/family put forth strong effort?
    (d) Are there co-occurring medical conditions that are complicating treatment? For example, co-occurring diabetes mellitus, celiac disease, or food allergies may make it difficult to increase food repertoire due to intolerance, allergy, or exaggerated fear of negative consequences of eating.
    (e) Are there co-occurring psychiatric conditions or behaviors that are complicating treatment? Co-occurring depression, anxiety, autism, substance use, or psychosis may impact appetite or involve behavioral challenges that make it difficult to increase intake.
    (f) Does the patient require medications (such as stimulants) that are adversely impacting appetite?
    (g) Are there factors or stresses at home that are affecting the family's ability to fully participate in treatment?

(h) How medically stable is the patient? Recent labs, growth charts, and subspecialty consultation reports may also help build a strong case for inpatient care.

3. What are the goals of hospitalization? Is the referring provider advocating for weaning someone off an NGT or G (gastric) tube? Hitting a goal weight? Working on increasing intake to hit a particular calorie level or expand food repertoire to include a wider range of foods? The more specific the ask, the better. Work with the treatment team and family to refine the goals of hospitalization to ensure that everyone is aligned.
4. Make sure to get authorization in writing and document names and positions of those involved in the process. Generally, it is best to have at least 1–2 weeks guaranteed. Ask about the process for requesting more time if needed. Typically, this is handled by case management/utilization review on the inpatient unit.

As ARFID becomes an increasingly mainstream diagnosis, more medical and mental health clinicians have been able to develop the skills needed to support them. However, many treatment deserts remain, and many patients have not had access to the appropriate treatment earlier in life. Not all treatment programs have the skills to develop customized programs for all needs. In these cases, intensive specialty programs may be necessary. Skilled referring providers can advocate with payors to help families access the appropriate treatment for a family's needs.

Chapter 12
Tube Feeding

At times, nasogastric tube (NGT) feeding may be indicated for a patient with ARFID. In this approach, a thin, flexible tube is inserted into the nostril such that liquid nutrition can be introduced directly into the stomach. Feeds can be administered in two main ways: continuous and bolus. Continuous feeds are provided by a pump giving a measured rate over several hours, while bolus feeds are often administered by gravity and given more quickly. Bolus feeds can approximate a meal, while continuous feeds are given much more slowly and may be useful in those experiencing a lot of GI symptoms. At one inpatient institution ARFID patients relied on more enteral nutrition and required longer hospitalizations than AN patients [1].

Within our treatment approach, tube feeding is usually not considered unless all other possibilities have first been tested. It can, however, be a tool to help a patient build their capacity to tolerate more nutrition when done in a step-by-step way that helps the patient gradually return to feeding by mouth. There are other instances, where tube feeding is needed for a longer duration of time because of a patient's limited capacity for feeding or due to a family's limited ability to support their required nutritional level.

Indications for NG Tube Feeding

ARFID- Fear of Aversive Consequences

With ARFID- fear of aversive consequences, efforts are made to avoid tube feeding since the patient at baseline is typically anxious about physical sensations. Rarely do these patients receive an NG tube on the first day of hospitalization unless it is requested. First, the patient will have supportive feeding sessions with the

A. B. Sinha et al., *Comprehensive Clinical Care for Adolescents with Avoidant/Restrictive Food Intake Disorder (ARFID)*,
https://doi.org/10.1007/978-3-031-92232-9_12

occupational therapist and nursing staff to see if their baseline nutrition can be progressed and if they can drink a supplement. Those with a fear of choking typically do not have difficulty drinking a supplement unless they struggle with the taste of the supplement (e.g., if they also have ARFID- sensory issues). For patients with a fear of vomiting, volume tolerance is usually the main barrier when consuming a supplement. If the oral nutrition progresses too slowly or the patient is showing significant signs of malnutrition (e.g. markedly low hearts or blood pressures), the medical team may initiate tube feeding to bolster their medical stability. Examples of this might include significant vitamin or electrolyte deficiencies that need immediate correction, or unstable vital signs. Additionally, the tube can help with medication management in cases where the patient has issues with pill swallowing or has a poor tolerance to oral medication. To help alleviate any anxiety around tube feeding, patients can benefit from starting on exclusive overnight feeds, at a moderate rate typically between 10 PM to 6 AM, to help promote the best possible tolerance and thus, success with enteral nutrition. Overnight tube feeding would allow the patient to be passively nourished while asleep and in a more relaxed state, and also would not significantly disrupt their daytime PO intake as they continue to work on their meal/snack progression with the help of the care team.

In some instances when there are overnight feeds, a patient may worry about eating an evening snack, since they fear they may get too full and vomit when the overnight feeds start. If this is the case, overnight feeds can start as early as 8:30 PM and replace the evening snack. Some patients do better if the feed is started while they are awake while others feel more comfortable with tube feeds starting while they are asleep. It is good to check in with the patient to see what they would feel the most comfortable with and then to observe what seems to work for that patient (e.g., if they are hypervigilant about when it starts, it is better to start while awake). Of note, patients typically complain of a poor appetite when overnight feeds end too close to breakfast. About 8 h of a nutrition break is typically helpful to stimulate an appetite in the morning. Therefore, overnight feeds and the subsequent meals are adjusted to accommodate for this. For example, if overnight feeds end at 6 AM, patients usually skip the morning meals and start with lunch as their first meal of the day. If overnight feeds end at 3 AM, patients can potentially have a late breakfast at 9 AM or opt for a mid-morning snack instead.

With a nutrition plan involving overnight feeds, usually patients are able to have some food during the day with the support of a behavior modification plan that helps promote increasing bites and overall portion sizes. This is typically done at structured meal and snack times. Often, a supplement is introduced at set intervals and the team works with the patient to gradually increase their capacity to drink the supplement as a replacement or as a method to meet their overall nutrition needs. As the patient progresses, options include: eating a specified amount of food, replacing the missing calories of the meal through the supplement or administering whatever replacement supplement could not be completed through the tube (often with a gravity bolus feed). As the patient demonstrates improvement in daytime nutrition, overnight feeds are gradually decreased until they no longer require overnight feeds. This may be done with or without the visual support of the Ladder Block Plan (see

OT chapter for details of the Ladder Block Plan). Typically these patients are completely weaned off of the NGT feeds prior to the hospital discharge. In the case where a more long-term tube feeding plan is needed for home, the care team will work with the family to establish a nutrition plan that can be replicated at home., Over time, the patient and family will continue to work on increasing oral intake and weaning the NG tube feeds.

Indications for Longer Term Tube Feeding and/or G-Tube Feeds

The longer a patient has had a fear of aversive consequences, the more time it may take to treat the fear. If the patient has been at a low weight for a sustained period and is not able to fully wean off the tube despite intervention, it can be helpful to consider a longer term tube feeding placement. This can "take the pressure off" from the daytime nutrition, which allows caregivers and the patient to explore increasing their PO intake at a more comfortable pace. With longer term tube feeding, it is essential for the patient and family to continue working closely with the treatment team to help the patient continue to build the skills that will be needed to wean off of the tube.

If the patient is continuing to make active progress, though slowly, it may be more appropriate to continue with an NG tube rather than moving to a gastric tube (G-tube), as they might eventually progress to the point where a tube is no longer required. However, if progress has stalled, the tube has been needed for over 6 months and likely will be required for at least a year, or if it is significantly disrupting activities of daily living (e.g., participation in school or other meaningful daily activities), it would be appropriate to consult with the surgical team to consider G-tube placement.

ARFID- Sensory Issues

Most ARFID patients with sensory issues can consume enough calories to maintain or gain weight when presented with an adequate amount of preferred foods. Caregivers can benefit from nutrition education that specifies how much preferred food is needed in order to maintain or promote weight gain. If tube feeding is indicated, it's usually because the patient's sensory issues are preventing them from getting enough of their required nutrients and/or calories to be medically/nutritionally safe. Micro- and macronutrient deficiencies can be a concern and if the patient has a very limited food repertoire. They may need to develop the capacity to take nutrition supplements by mouth in addition to developing the skill of expanding their food repertoire. Usually individuals with ARFID- sensory issues have had this eating pattern for many years, if not their entire life. It's important to set the expectation that changes are often slow and it may take months to make meaningful change.Despite this, with structure and motivation, it is often possible.

Anytime NG tube feeds are initiated, the care team will continue to focus on how to best promote oral intake and thus, wean the tube. For example, if tube feeding is initiated to address a protein deficit, the team would focus on ways to support the patient in getting enough protein. Often a daytime supplement would be started in a small capacity, with step-by-step efforts to increase quantity over time.

ARFID- Low Interest

Many ARFID patients who were considered in the past to have failure to thrive or lifelong low interest have spent years on a low growth curve. Typically these patients start to deviate from their usual growth curve into a much lower growth curve, sometimes below the 5th percentile and off the chart completely once puberty hits. They often struggle to keep up with the increased nutrition demands common to entering puberty.

These patients struggle to find value or joy in eating, have no favorite foods, or struggle with the stamina to keep eating when feeling too full. Therefore, short-term or long-term NG tube feeds may be considered to support their growth and height potential during the critical developmental years.

In cases where long-term tube feeding (typically with a G-tube) has been initiated, patients typically receive overnight feeds to avoid disrupting their daily activities (school, sports).When working with individuals who are interested in weaning after chronic G tube use, the goal remains the same: to gradually increase daytime nutrition while decreasing overnight feeds. Once they are able to demonstrate adequate growth and medical stability, for at least three or more months, G tube removal can be considered.

Sometimes during hospitalization, an NG-tube is used for a short period to help the body get more quickly accustomed to the required nutritional level. Keeping an NG tube may motivate them to eat more due to the inconvenience (physically or socially) of having an NG tube, and may allow the patient to avoid surgical G tube placement.

Using the Ladder Block Plan in NG Tube Feeding

The Ladder Block Plan (LBP) can be a powerful tool in supporting an increase in daytime nutrition and wean from an NG tube as it provides a detailed visual examination of patient progress. Please see Chap. 8 for background and a full description of the Ladder Block Plan. In general, the LBP can be useful in the following situations:

- There is a goal of weaning off tube feeds
- The patient is consistently taking 1000 calories or more by mouth
- The patient is able to drink 2 oz. of a supplement by mouth at meals and snacks
- Parent is interested in using the plan and willing to support it's use
- There is a member of the multidisciplinary team available to support moving and modifying the blocks of the ladder block plan to increase intake

Sample Scenario: This scenario includes a patient exhibited weaning off overnight NG tube feeds. Their best overall PO caloric intake the day before the Ladder Block Plan was initiated. Therefore, this day's caloric intake was used to determine the block value (Table 12.1). This patient's goal calories are 3000 calories/day and currently this patient is taking in 1020 calories by mouth.

Overnight feeds: 2000 kcals
Mid Morning snack: 95 kcals
Lunch: 285 kcals
Afternoon Snack: 126 kcals
Dinner: 293 kcals
Night Snack: 221 kcals

The below ladder block plan [12.1] that was created initially based on 1020 kcals/block.

Table 12.1 Demonstration of how to apply the ladder block plan formula using a sample scenario with a resulting ladder block plan (Fig 12.1)

Meals	Day 3 (highest of past 3 days	Meal kcals/ quotient	Resulting answer to determine # of blocks	Blocks/ meal per formula	Resulting calories/block and total if keeping value the same	Resulting calories/block if advancing calories by 100 kcals that day
Formula for Caloric value/block					1020/10 = 102 kcal/block	1120/10 = 112 kcal/block
AM snack kcals	95	95/102	0.93=	1 blocks	1 blocks = 102 kcals	1 blocks = 112 kcal
Lunch kcals	285	285/102	2.79=	3 blocks	3 blocks = 306 kcal	3 blocks = 336 kcal
Afternoon snack kcals	126	126/102	1.24=	1 block	1 block = 102 kcal	1 block = 112 kcal
Dinner kcals	293	293/102	2.87=	3 blocks	3 blocks = 306 kcal	3 blocks = 336 kcal
Night snack kcals	221	221/102	2.16=	2 block	2 block = 204 kcal	2 blocks = 224 kcal
Cumulative value	1020			10 blocks	1020 kcals 102 kcal/block 10 blocks	1120 kcal 112 kcal/block 10 blocks

LADDER BLOCK PLAN

Sheet to track meeting nutritional needs to support brain and body optimal function

Day:	Day:	Day:	Day:	Day:	Day:	Day:
Used strategies	Used strategies	Used strategies	Used strategies	Used strategies	Used strategies	Used strategies
All green	All green	All green	All green	All green	All green	All green
All met	All met	All met	All met	All met	All met	All met
PM Snack	PM Snack	PM Snack	PM Snack	PM Snack	PM Snack	PM Snack
PM Snack	PM Snack	PM Snack	PM Snack	PM Snack	PM Snack	PM Snack
Dinner	Dinner	Dinner	Dinner	Dinner	Dinner	Dinner
Dinner	Dinner	Dinner	Dinner	Dinner	Dinner	Dinner
Dinner	Dinner	Dinner	Dinner	Dinner	Dinner	Dinner
Snack	Snack	Snack	Snack	Snack	Snack	Snack
Lunch	Lunch	Lunch	Lunch	Lunch	Lunch	Lunch
Lunch	Lunch	Lunch	Lunch	Lunch	Lunch	Lunch
Lunch	Lunch	Lunch	Lunch	Lunch	Lunch	Lunch
AM Snack	AM Snack	AM Snack	AM Snack	AM Snack	AM Snack	AM Snack
Extra kcals:	Extra kcals:	Extra kcals:	Extra kcals:	Extra kcals:	Extra kcals:	Extra kcals:

- Each meal/ snack block represents a specific nutritional amount per RD guidelines of specific caloric value/ block.
- Please color block Green when completed at meal PO and coloring yellow when completed at a later time
- Please note that coloring the full amount in green represents getting all required nutrition at that mealtime with any nutritional source PO.
- Food items may be exchanged or replaced with other food items or supplement (if desired).
- It is important to keep rotating food items to avoid food jags.
- If more kcals are achieved during a meal than the block needs, record the extra value in the bottom "extra kcal" section, they may be used to complete later blocks as needed/desired (within the same day only).
- Only color in complete block(s) if that full nutritional value is consumed at that meal or used in combination with the "extra kcal" calories. When those are used, cross them off to indicate they have been utilized.
- Always first color the blocks for that meal/ snack before making up nutrition from a prior meal.
- Please document points for each meal and snack.

Fig. 12.1 Ladder Block Plan example used an NG tube feeding wean with an initial step-b-step in PO nutrition as documented on the Ladder Block Plan (LBP) Nasogastric tube (NGT) feeding

In this particular ladder block plan, the plan is only showing the daily by mouth nutritional goals as indicated in the blocks. It is recommended that these goals are gradually increased. When the patient exceeds the by-mouth nutritional goals, it is recommended that the value of each block is increased the subsequent day. For example, if the patient's goal was 1020 kcals with a 10 block plan, but they took in 1105 calories (usually a calorie count is kept to determine this) and the goal was to advance by 95 kcals, it is recommended to round that to 1200 divided by 10 blocks with a block value of 120 calories/block. (Goal calories should be divisible by the number of blocks, resulting in an integer). However, if the patient is increasing their nutrition only at dinner time, a half block or 1 block might be added for the dinner period.

In a different scenario, if the patient is not exceeding their blocks but they are hitting their goals for 1–2 day, increase the daily nutrition by 100 calories. To do this, add 100 to the goal calories (in this case 100+ 1020 = 1120 divided by 10 blocks = 112 calories/block). Now, the blocks below are set up at 112 kcal/block which is an increase in daytime nutrition by an extra 100 calories by mouth. The medical team would likely decrease the night time nutrition by the same amount (or more) to encourage by-mouth nutrition. As the daytime nutrition is increased decrease the overnight nutrition y at least the same amount (potentially decrease more to increase appetite). While decreasing calories may hinder weight progress, it does speed up the weaning process.

If the patient is not hitting their goals, do not increase the caloric value per block. Instead, work with the patient to further explore and move through barriers.

There are times where the Ladder Block Plan can mimic an eat-replace-NG model plan (Fig. 12.2) (see Nutrition chapter 5 for full details of eat and replace model). The patient eats as much as they can and then drinks the replacement supplement. Whatever they do not drink is then placed through the NG tube immediately after the meal using a gravity bolus feed. This allows individuals to acclimate to appropriate volumes of nutrition during typical mealtimes.

For example, if the patient was taking 1000 calories overnight and 1000 calories by day, initially the ladder block may change to just increasing the daytime calories by 100 calories so that the offer to drink it versus getting it through the NG-tube may seem more appealing. The overnight feed can gradually be decreased with increased day time PO expectations by step-by-step increasing the block value or block placement as the patient progresses in the amount of nutrition taken by mouth.

LADDER BLOCK PLAN

Sheet to track meeting nutritional needs to support brain and body optimal function

Monday	Tuesday	Wednesday	Thursday	Friday	Saturday	Sunday
Used strategies	Used strategies	Used strategies	Used strategies	Used strategies	Used strategies	Used strategies
All green	All green	All green	All green	All green	All green	All green
All met	All met	All met	All met	All met	All met	All met
Snack	Snack	Snack	Snack	Snack	Snack	Snack
Snack	Snack	Snack	Snack	Snack	Snack	Snack
Dinner	Dinner	Dinner	Dinner	Dinner	Dinner	Dinner
Dinner	Dinner	Dinner	Dinner	Dinner	Dinner	Dinner
Dinner	Dinner	Dinner	Dinner	Dinner	Dinner	Dinner
Snack	Snack	Snack	Snack	Snack	Snack	Snack
Snack	Snack	Snack	Snack	Snack	Snack	Snack
Lunch	Lunch	Lunch	Lunch	Lunch	Lunch	Lunch
Lunch	Lunch	Lunch	Lunch	Lunch	Lunch	Lunch
AM snack	AM snack	AM snack	AM snack	AM snack	AM snack	AM snack
Extra kcals:	Extra kcals:	Extra kcals:	Extra kcals:	Extra kcals:	Extra kcals:	Extra kcals:

- Each meal/ snack block represents "a block of nutrition" per RD guidelines
- Please color block Green when completed at meal through food or supplement completed by mouth
- If supplement is completed by NG tube, please color in gray
- Please note that coloring the full amount in green represents getting all required nutrition at that mealtime with any nutritional source.
- Food items may be exchanged or replaced with other food items or suppliment (if desired)
- It is important to keep rotating food items to avoid food jags
- If more kcals are achieved during a meal than the block needs, record the extra value in the bottom "extra kcal" section, they may be used to complete later blocks as needed/desired (within the same day only)
- Only color in complete block(s) if that full nutritional value is consumed at that meal or used in combination with the "extra kcal" calories. When those are used, cross them off to indicate they have been utilized.

Fig. 12.2 Sample eat-replace-NG Ladder Block Plan used in advancement of a NG tube feed wean

> Step-by-step the expectations for day-time nutrition can be increased (as the patient progresses in by-mouth nutrition) and night time overnight feed decreased until all nutrition is achieved by day. It is best to keep the NG-tube in place until the patient has achieved 3 days of 100% by-mouth feeds or until they ask for it out while achieving the desired nutrition (whichever comes first).

There are occasions when older patients benefit from seeing a visual on the ladder block plan of the blocks that they are receiving overnight versus in the day time so that their progress feels clearer. If a patient would benefit from seeing this visually, it is possible to set a long-term goal of what the ladder block plan would look like and color in the parts that are scheduled for overnight in gray. This can be done in 1 of 2 ways, either coloring in the components from each meal that would occur at night (Fig. 12.3) or having a separate section for night time nutrition (Fig. 12.4). See the below examples of samples of 3000 calorie goals. For the below, each block = 300 kcals. It is likely as the patient progresses that some blocks will need to be adapted to 1/2 block values.

For some patients it can be highly motivating to see the level of gray decreasing and the level of daytime green increasing. Patients achieve the "all green" goal when they have gotten all nutrition by mouth during the day at the specified time.

LADDER BLOCK PLAN

Sheet to track meeting nutritional needs to support brain and body optimal function

Monday	Tuesday	Wednesday	Thursday	Friday	Saturday	Sunday
Used strategies	Used strategies	Used strategies	Used strategies	Used strategies	Used strategies	Used strategies
All green	All green	All green	All green	All green	All green	All green
All met	All met	All met	All mot	All met	All met	All met
Snack	Snack	Snack	Snack	Snack	Snack	Snack
Snack	Snack	Snack	Snack	Snack	Snack	Snack
Dinner	Dinner	Dinner	Dinner	Dinner	Dinner	Dinner
Dinner	Dinner	Dinner	Dinner	Dinner	Dinner	Dinner
Dinner	Dinner	Dinner	Dinner	Dinner	Dinner	Dinner
Snack	Snack	Snack	Snack	Snack	Snack	Snack
Snack	Snack	Snack	Snack	Snack	Snack	Snack
Lunch	Lunch	Lunch	Lunch	Lunch	Lunch	Lunch
Lunch	Lunch	Lunch	Lunch	Lunch	Lunch	Lunch
AM snack	AM snack	AM snack	AM snack	AM snack	AM snack	AM snack
Extra kcals:	Extra kcals:	Extra kcals:	Extra kcals:	Extra kcals:	Extra kcals:	Extra kcals:

- Each meal/ snack block represents "a block of nutrition" per RD guidelines
- Please color block Green when completed at meal, Yellow when completed at a later meal
- Note that nutrition that gray blocks are used to demo where nutrition that is currently received overnight will be in the future
- Please note that coloring the full amount in green represents getting all required nutrition at that mealtime with any nutritional source.
- Food items may be exchanged or replaced with other food items or suppliment (if desired)
- It is important to keep rotating food items to avoid food jags
- If more kcals are achieved during a meal than the block needs, record the extra value in the bottom "extra kcal" section, they may be used to complete later blocks as needed/desired (within the same day only)
- Only color in complete block(s) if that full nutritional value is consumed at that meal or used in combination with the "extra kcal" calories. When those are used, cross them off to indicate they have been utilized.
- If blocks are not fully completed at any meal, color only up to what has been completed, leaving that section blank, if made up later (by going over at a subsequent meal or snack and giving caloric credit), color in yellow.
- Always first color the blocks for that meal/ snack before making up nutrition from a prior meal.

Fig. 12.3 Ladder Block Plan that shows goal blocks with NG nutrition in gray, sued for advancement of an NG tube feeding wean

LADDER BLOCK PLAN

Sheet to track meeting nutritional needs to support brain and body optimal function

Monday	Tuesday	Wednesday	Thursday	Friday	Saturday	Sunday
Used strategies	Used strategies	Used strategies	Used strategies	Used strategies	Used strategies	Used strategies
All green	All green	All green	All green	All green	All green	All green
All met	All met	All met	All met	All met	All met	All met
Overnight	Overnight	Overnight	Overnight	Overnight	Overnight	Overnight
Overnight	Overnight	Overnight	Overnight	Overnight	Overnight	Overnight
Overnight	Overnight	Overnight	Overnight	Overnight	Overnight	Overnight
Overnight	Overnight	Overnight	Overnight	Overnight	Overnight	Overnight
Overnight	Overnight	Overnight	Overnight	Overnight	Overnight	Overnight
Overnight	Overnight	Overnight	Overnight	Overnight	Overnight	Overnight
Snack	Snack	Snack	Snack	Snack	Snack	Snack
Dinner	Dinner	Dinner	Dinner	Dinner	Dinner	Dinner
Snack	Snack	Snack	Snack	Snack	Snack	Snack
Lunch	Lunch	Lunch	Lunch	Lunch	Lunch	Lunch
AM snack	AM snack	AM snack	AM snack	AM snack	AM snack	AM snack
Extra kcals:	Extra kcals:	Extra kcals:	Extra kcals:	Extra kcals:	Extra kcals:	Extra kcals:

- Each meal/ snack block represents "a block of nutrition" per RD guidelines
- Please color block Green when completed at meal, Yellow when completed at a later meal
- Note that nutrition that gray blocks are currently received overnight and in the future will be moved to meal and snack times
- Please note that coloring the full amount in green represents getting all required nutrition at that mealtime with any nutritional source.
- Food items may be exchanged or replaced with other food items or suppliment (if desired)
- It is important to keep rotating food items to avoid food jags
- If more kcals are achieved during a meal than the block needs, record the extra value in the bottom "extra kcal" section, they may be used to complete later blocks as needed/desired (within the same day only)
- Only color in complete block(s) if that full nutritional value is consumed at that meal or used in combination with the "extra kcal" calories. When those are used, cross them off to indicate they have been utilized.
- If blocks are not fully completed at any meal, color only up to what has been completed, leaving that section blank, if made up later (by going over at a subsequent meal or snack and giving caloric credit), color in yellow.
- Always first color the blocks for that meal/ snack before making up nutrition from a prior meal.

Fig. 12.4 Ladder Block Plan that shows overnight nutrition in gray, used for advancement of an NG tube feeding wean

Conclusion

When possible, it is optimal to avoid tube feeding in ARFID patients. However, when the NG tube is needed it can be a tool for weight gain and nutritional progress. When this tool is simultaneously paired with treatment that supports improving by mouth nutrition, the NG tube can assist the patient in building the tolerance for a higher caloric volume. Additionally, when the patient cannot eat enough consistently to support their health, or the family is truly not able to support sufficient feeding, a feeding tube may be the most ethical choice in ensuring that a patient meets their developmental potential.

Reference

1. Strandjord SE, Sieke EH, Richmond M, Rome ES. Avoidant/restrictive food intake disorder: illness and hospital course in patients hospitalized for nutritional insufficiency. J Adolesc Health. 2015;57(6):673–8. https://doi.org/10.1016/j.jadohealth.2015.08.003.

Chapter 13
Preparing to Transition to Adulthood (College or Otherwise)

The transition to adulthood is an exciting, yet stressful, time for even the most well-adjusted individual. Late adolescence is a developmental stage marked by several biopsychosocial changes. The frontal lobe is continuing to myelinate and mature up until around age 25–30, leading to improvements in impulsivity and executive function. Major psychological tasks during this phase include the processes of separation and individuation from one's family of origin, as well as further developing and cementing one's identity and learning to live independently. Many young people in this age range do not have experience managing all the activities of daily living on their own. Often, parents find themselves enforcing bedtime and morning wake-up, monitoring school attendance, scheduling activities, making medical appointments, and refilling and administering medications up until high school graduation. Budgeting, laundry, and grocery shopping are additional tasks that many young adults do not have experience with prior to moving out of the family home. The degree to which parents were providing structure and support is often not fully evident until the youth starts living independently [1].

Paths to adulthood after high school are varied and can include taking a gap year, entering the military or volunteer corps service, entry into the workforce, or transition to college or university studies. Post-secondary education is increasingly common, and youth with previously diagnosed mental health conditions have been able to attend college at higher rates than in the past, likely owing to increased identification and treatment earlier in life. These individuals need strong transition from pediatric to adult mental health services, which can be challenging due to differences in philosophy between pediatric and adult care. Child and adolescent mental health treatment is typically systems focused, with parents, schools, pediatricians, and coaches actively encouraged to be involved in care. Systems often work together to communicate and support an individual even when motivation for treatment wanes. Adult mental health is typically more focused on the autonomy of the individual, with the belief that the patient needs to want and accept the interventions

A. B. Sinha et al., *Comprehensive Clinical Care for Adolescents with Avoidant/Restrictive Food Intake Disorder (ARFID)*,
https://doi.org/10.1007/978-3-031-92232-9_13

recommended. Individuals frequently fall through the cracks when making the transition to adult services, because providers are unlikely to let parents or other systems know that they are not following through with care [2].

Colleges and universities have mental health services available through their student health and counseling centers, but there is no standardization regarding the kinds of services available. Some universities offer a limited number of sessions before referring students out to local providers. Others limit interventions to counseling related to homesickness, roommate challenges, and career counseling and stipulate that more chronic and serious conditions need to be treated off campus [3]. Those needing academic accommodations in the high school setting will need to seek out similar services in the university setting. Whereas the onus to identify and provide services to children and teens is the responsibility of the school under K-12 education law, this responsibility shifts to the adult patient in the university setting, and is covered by the Americans with Disabilities Act laws instead [4]. It is imperative that families investigate the available resources early in the college application and decision-making process so there are no surprises along the way. It behooves families to consider things like the level of medical and psychiatric stability in place at the time of transition and the young adult's willingness to access mental health support when deciding where to go to school. Is this a rural or urban campus? Are there appropriate mental health supports nearby? How far away are family and/or trusted adults if there is a crisis? How much oversight and support are needed? How frequently can parents visit? While tempting, parents cannot rely on roommates, faculty, or other peers to monitor and notify them of concerns.

Things for families to keep in mind while making decisions about college:

- Location (urban or rural, proximity to home or other friends/family)
- Availability of appropriate medical and mental health treatment (likely to be highly dependent on location). How many sessions will they be able to access? Will they be referred off campus for chronic needs?
- Is there a strong office of accessible education (disability office) to help develop a plan for academic accommodations? Is the student motivated to access those accommodations? What paperwork is necessary to request accommodations? Start this process early to be sure there are no delays that might adversely impact academic success early on.
- How medically and psychiatrically stable is the student? Do they understand their diagnoses and medical/psychiatric needs? Do they understand the target and potential adverse side effects of the medications they take?
- How independent is the student at baseline? Are they requiring high levels of support from parents to complete activities of daily living and medical care?
- Are they ready? Might they be in a more stable position if they took a gap year, or if they started out living at home and attending community college to practice balancing the rigors of school while having some scaffolding in place to help them become more independent? Often, parents want their children to "stay in step" with their peers, but delaying the transition may well optimize chances of success.

Youth with ARFID frequently need additional planning to successfully navigate the transition to adulthood. This is especially true of those who also have co-occurring conditions requiring additional medical and/or psychiatric care. Those with chronic low interest/appetite and those with long term selective eating are uniquely vulnerable to backsliding into old habits and patterns of eating when making the transition to living independently. They may need extra practice creating internal structure in their schedules to make sure that they are able to eat even when they are not hungry, or when something unexpected happens and they are not able to access food easily at designated mealtimes. This may mean having supplies of shelf stable food at the ready in their residence hall rooms, cars, or backpacks so they always have a backup plan. Families need to be aware of the usual policies and procedures around campus meal plans. Must the student live on campus and have a meal plan (even if they don't like the food available in the cafeteria)? What will they do on weekends or holidays when dining halls are potentially closed or open for shorter periods of time during the day? What if they sleep through breakfast and lunch? Are they allowed to have a refrigerator and/or microwave in their room? How will they resist the temptations of staying up late, playing video games, and ignoring the alarm clock each morning?

Beyond creating structure and support, families need to consider oversight and how they will know whether their student is staying healthy and balanced. It is wise to work out an agreement well in advance of making the transition to school so that expectations are clear. While young adults have the legal ability to make their own decisions, most of them are reliant on their parents for emotional and financial support. Parents cannot force a loved one over the age of 18 into treatment, but they can link ongoing financial support (including car insurance, cell phone fees, and tuition) to ongoing physical and mental health and stability. Often, families find it beneficial to work with treatment teams well in advance of the transition to college to determine a treatment contract. Such contracts are most helpful when they lay out clear expectations of the minimal parameters needed to remain enrolled. Parents also need to be honest about what they are willing to enforce, as contracts are not particularly useful when the contingencies are not followed [3].

Elements of a treatment contract:

- Define diagnoses and their treatment needs. Is everyone aligned on the issue and recommended interventions?
- Who is on the treatment team, and what are their roles?
- How often must the student meet with each team member? What happens if they avoid scheduling appointments, late cancel, or no show? It can help to stipulate that the student needs to make, attend, and participate in all appointments, and agrees to follow the medical interventions recommended.
- Does the student need to sign a release of information for each team member? What kind of information may the team member share with parents?
- What are the parameters for remaining enrolled in school (stable weight, vital signs, participation in treatment sessions)?

- Who is responsible for making the call about the need for additional medical intervention?
- Who makes the decision about the need to withdraw from school?
- If a medical leave occurs, what are the parameters for return to school?

Families often struggle with how much information to share with a university about a student's mental health needs out of concern about undue oversight or stigma. This is ultimately a family decision, but it may be helpful for families to keep in mind that universities are motivated to keep students happy, healthy, and in a position to graduate. Most are incredibly supportive and willing to work with families to find solutions wherever possible to allow students to remain safely enrolled [4].

Transition to adulthood is an invigorating yet stressful time, and making this transition in the setting of chronic medical and mental health conditions can be overwhelming. Families supporting a young adult with ARFID will benefit from thoughtful planning that occurs well in advance of navigating this transition, and treatment providers working with eating disorders need to be fully apprised of how best to support them.

References

1. Chan V, Derenne J, editors. Transition-age youth mental health care: bridging the gap between pediatric and adult psychiatric care. Springer; 2021.
2. Martel A, Derenne J, Leebens PK, editors. Promoting safe and effective transitions to college for youth with mental health conditions: a case-based guide to best practices. Springer; 2018.
3. Derenne JL. Successfully launching adolescents with eating disorders to college: the child and adolescent psychiatrist's perspective. J Am Acad Child Adolesc Psychiatry. 2013;52(6):559–61.
4. Derenne J. Eating disorders in transitional age youth. Child Adolesc Psychiatr Clin N Am. 2019;28(4):567–72.

Part II
Case-Based Chapters

Chapter 14
Sensory Inpatient Case Study (Nick)

Case Presentation

Nick is a 12-year-old cisgender male, born at 34 weeks' gestation, with a longstanding history of poor PO intake and growth. Due to his failure to thrive, he has had multiple subspecialty evaluations, including with GI and Endocrinology, who attributed his growth delay to behavioral issues.

Notable feeding history includes delayed initiation of solid foods at 18 months due to parental concern about frequent spitting out of food. At age 12 years, he continues to prefer liquids to solids, although he enjoys food from certain fast-food restaurants. He endorses wanting to gain weight and denies any body image concerns.

In a routine well child check visit with his PCP, Nick is noted to have continued low weight with minimal weight gain from his prior year's well-check appointment (Fig. 14.1). He is also found to be hypotensive. He is referred to the inpatient medical unit for stabilization and management.

Notable studies include: Bone age compatible with that of a 10 year old male.

A. B. Sinha et al., *Comprehensive Clinical Care for Adolescents with Avoidant/Restrictive Food Intake Disorder (ARFID)*,
https://doi.org/10.1007/978-3-031-92232-9_14

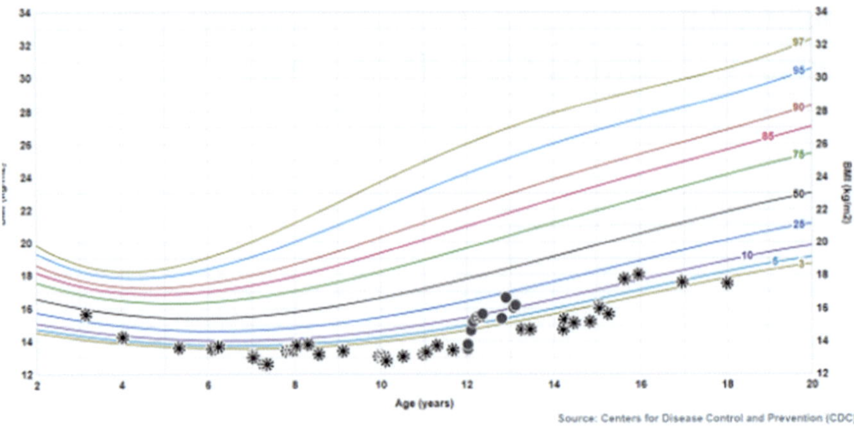

Fig. 14.1 Growth chart for Nick

Medical

Nick presented to the hospital with medical instability of hypotension, severe malnutrition, and lack of appropriate weight gain. Prior to admission, he had received subspecialty care to evaluate his low weight; all available notes and laboratory values were reviewed to ensure a thorough evaluation had been completed to rule out any other etiologies to weight loss that might explain Nick's more chronic difficulty in gaining and maintaining weight. Typically, evaluations performed more than a year or two prior to admission may need to be repeated to ensure new issues have not developed (such as repeating thyroid studies).

During Nick's admission, the medical team monitored his vital signs which stabilized with improvements in his nutrition. As his vital signs improved, he was able to increase his physical activity from being on bedrest to being able to walk within the hospital unit. Electrolytes were also monitored for refeeding syndrome with measurements performed daily for the first several days, then becoming less frequent. Nick did not have any electrolyte changes during his admission.

During his admission, parents wondered about his "ideal" weight and height, noting that he is shorter than many of his peers. For patients with chronic eating issues, it is not unusual to see height, in addition to weight, affected. His bone age, performed prior to his admission, showed an estimated age of 10 years (2 years less than his chronologic age). It can be challenging to determine growth goals for individuals who may have chronic malnutrition and subsequent stunting of growth. The height goal can be based on the mid-parental height with the incorporation of the calculated standard deviation. Often, a BMI goal will be set as the highest of two options: highest percentile reached in the past or the tenth percentile. The bone age will not be used in calculating the overall goal height or BMI, but can help estimate the window of time remaining for potential catch-up height if nutrition is able to be normalized and maintained. For Nick, given his bone age, his window for growth was significant. Given the chronicity of his lower BMI, an initial goal BMI was set for him as between the tenth and 25th percentile.

Psychiatry

Nick's parents indicated that Nick had lifelong symptoms of selective eating, accompanied by low appetite and diminished interest in eating. Because he appeared to be so upset and dysregulated by the experience of trying new foods and eating, parents had accommodated negative behavior for years. He had similar meltdowns when frustrated or disappointed in non-food related settings. They felt bad for him and didn't want him to be distressed, so they allowed him to consume whatever he wanted, at any time. This led to parents feeling burned out and stressed, with both feeling like short order cooks at all times of the day.

In the same way that Nick was motivated to eat and gain weight, parents were motivated to do whatever they could to support him. Psychology worked mostly with the parents on parent management training techniques that would generalize to other settings. They reviewed the concept of a behavioral extinction burst, which sometimes happens in response to parents making changes and being firmer. In an extinction burst, a child or teen starts to escalate unwanted behaviors in the hopes that parents will give in. A classic example is a child having a temper tantrum in the aisle of a store, in hopes that the parent will buy them a toy. Parents who are tired or embarrassed may sometimes give in to stop the tantrum, but in doing so run the risk of encouraging unhelpful behavior in the future. They also reviewed strategies for managing their own stress and dysregulation in these situations, which they noted allowed them to be more calm, firm, and consistent in their limit setting. Nick's parents were able to stay consistent with expectations, and even though there was a little pushback, Nick ultimately realized that parents weren't going to give in, and behavior improved.

Nick had been started on cyproheptadine by his pediatrician with limited benefit. The team discussed the need to increase his appetite and interest in food. Mirtazapine was briefly considered given that he had some anxiety and nausea during the renourishment process. However, given the need to jumpstart his progress quickly (due to being hospitalized), the decision was made to start a low dose atypical antipsychotic. Ultimately, he started on aripiprazole at 1 mg daily (which was titrated up to 2 mg daily) as parents were concerned about fatigue during the day and the potential for oversedation on other medications in this class. Baseline metabolic monitoring laboratory studies were obtained, including a lipid panel, hemoglobin A1C, and prolactin.

Nutrition

During the initial nutrition assessment, Nick and his parents collaborated on completing the 5 Food Guide to color code his food preferences. Nick was a selective eater with immature oral motor skills, so he gravitated towards liquids, soft foods such as soups or oatmeal, or some home cooked Indian meals such as Mom's curry and paratha.

Nick typically ate three meals per day, but breakfast most often consisted of only one to two items (bread with butter) or a smoothie. Lunch at school was limited since he disliked most food offered at school; he sometimes would eat a slice of pizza or would have a banana with potato chips. Dinners were the biggest meal since they were at home with his family, and typically consisted of Indian cuisine made by his mother. Snacks were either yogurt or fresh fruit.

Parents were shocked by Nick's estimated calorie and weight goals. Upon admission, Nick's caloric intake was at least 1000 calories less than his goal, explaining why Nick had minimal yearly weight gain since age nine. Nick's hospital nutrition plan first consisted of a 1600 kcal/day individualized meal plan that provided three meals and two snacks per day. His meal plan provided his preferred foods (green) and occasionally some neutral foods (yellow). Each meal had a liquid or soft item to help make eating easier. Nick was volume restricted and had been used to smaller meals his entire life. He needed time to gradually expand his stomach. Therefore, energy density was key. Also, he was selective but not necessarily fearful of new foods, so food chaining was implemented right away. The RD looked for any trends in the foods he liked or gravitated towards and started the food chaining process by providing foods that were similar to his current preferred foods. For example, since Nick liked chocolate and cookies, parents were asked to bring in chocolate filled biscuit cookies. Later, the RD asked Nick to eat cookies with chocolate ice cream which eventually led to him trying cookies and cream ice cream. Parents were very willing to provide outside foods. The RD brainstormed with parents on what foods they can bring in to complement the foods offered by the hospital. As Nick is ethnically and culturally Indian and his parents served traditional homemade foods, the RD worked to include his typically consumed foods into his inpatient meal plan while being nutritionally monitored.

Over time, Nick was able to tolerate the meal plan quite well until his daily caloric increases reached his estimated calorie goal of 2400 kcal/day. At this higher meal plan, he then started to rely more on liquid replacement to meet his full nutritional needs. With more food presented on his plate, he did his best with keeping up with the volume but would often feel fatigued by the end of the meal.

The above chart (Fig. 14.2) shows the amount of nutrition needed to reach Nick's caloric daily goal of 2400 kcal/day. His meals/snacks incorporated some cultural, home cooked foods and in red font are the challenge food items he needed to try for exposure. Nick was encouraged to eat as much as he could of the challenge food items but was not expected to consume replacement if he were unable to consume it all. Some of the challenge foods were ones that Nick agreed to try and some were

	Challenge Food Items in RED: NOT part of meal plan. No replacement needed.								
DAY		DATE		2400 KCALS					
Breakfast		Lunch		Snack		Dinner		Snack	
Hardboiled Egg (2)	160	FROM HOME: Shrimp Curry (1.5 cups)	350	FROM HOME: Rainbow Goldfish (1 package)	120	Chicken Quesadilla (1 whole)	407	FROM HOME: Fruit Gushers (1 pouch)	90
Oatmeal (3/4 cup)	110	FROM HOME: Roti (1.5 pieces)	125	Banana (1 whole)	100	Chicken Noodle Soup (6 oz)	120	Whole Milk (8 oz)	160
Whole Milk (8 oz)	160	Jasmine Rice (1/3 cup)	70	Blueberry Yogurt (6 oz)	140	Vanilla Ice Cream Cup (1/2 cup)	130	Mixed Nuts (1 oz)	
Canned Pears (1/2 cup)	60	Apple Juice (4 oz)	60	Popsicle (1)		Carrot Sticks (8 each)	28		
Pork Sausage (1 link)		Seasoned Broccoli (1/2 cup)	27			Julienne Vegetable Blend (1/4 cup)			
		Fresh Pineapple (1 cup)							
	490		632		360		685		250
								2417	

Fig. 14.2 Sample meal plan for Nick

ones that were chosen by the RD, based on what Nick could potentially like and what was available from the hospital kitchen at the time.

While the meal plan continued to increase, parents expressed concern about his continued need for replacement. The team explained that his reliance on replacement was expected and likely necessary at this time. With less food presented, Nick was more likely to eat a larger percentage of the food. However, as the food portions increased, Nick was limited by satiety, and thus, was unable to complete everything and needed to rely on replacement more. The RD reassured parents that this normally happens in the beginning of renourishment but is eventually tackled as a nutrition goal, usually after the patient has been weight restored.

In 2 weeks, Nick was able to eat more solid food, tolerate increased volumes, incorporate more exposure foods, and gain a total of six pounds during his admission, exceeding his parents' expectations. Nick and his family learned the skills needed to provide an adequate nutrition plan that balanced homemade cultural foods, foods Nick preferred, and foods Nick needed to try in order to continue the food repertoire expansion work.

Upon discharge from the hospital, Nick's eating and intake continued to improve and he continued to incorporate recommendations into his home routine. His eating speed improved (though was still slower than many) when he was made aware of his pacing. Importantly, he gained weight and his family was able to see that with support and adequate nutrition he could exhibit growth and continue weight gain .

Occupational Therapy

Nick reported a strong desire to gain weight- 10/10 and his willingness to work at it was also a 10/10. Nick demonstrated chronic hypersensitivity to texture and taste, excessive chewing, food pocketing, immature chewing patterns with some foods, and poor attention to meals. All these factors led to meals frequently lasting more than an hour. Nick's delayed introduction to solids at 8 months created a huge disadvantage for oral motor skills as development of eating and chewing were delayed due to lack of exposure. This likely is responsible for his preference for liquids over solids, his inability to consume more than a very small portion of food items, and his refusal to eat anything with an intact skin.

Occupational therapy interventions taught prior to the first meal observation included techniques for dealing with fullness (Happy Valley Point, Chap. 7, Fig. 7.2) and nausea (N6, see Chap. 7, Fig. 7.1). A Reliefband trial was initiated to address nausea (see Chap. 7, techniques for nausea). During the first meal, Nick tended to chew all his food on his right side, which increased his overall chewing time. He took very large bites and chewed excessively, pocketing his food in his cheek. He often would bring his knee(s) to his chest while eating and was redirected to use upright posture with his back supported with a pillow and feet flat on the ground for all meals. The OT also observed that Nick was hesitant to try new foods. Since he preferred liquids, he was able to drink full replacement for missed nutrition within 5–10 min.

Since he was able to drink easily and liked the available nutrition supplement, he was placed on an eat and replace plan. His feeding plan allowed him the opportunity to swap out food items for preferred ones, which ultimately helped meet his energy needs and he required less replacement. A food exploration log was introduced, and Nick was encouraged to use it for all newer foods (see Chap. 7, Chap. 22). He was advised to eat new food items at the beginning of the meal, and started practicing taking more moderate bites and swallowing sooner rather than pocketing his food.

Nick's mother privately expressed concerns about using the supplement to replace missed nutrition. The OT reviewed that Nick's oral motor skills were immature and that the first goal was getting enough nutrition since his bone-age was delayed and he was at a low height and weight for his age. She was happy that he was eating something at each meal and snack, taking liquid supplements, and gaining weight. This surprised his mother as she believed it was very difficult for him to gain weight. The OT collaboratively developed an incentive behavioral modification plan with the parents and got Nick's buy in as well. The reward chosen was a monetary reward and he was able to earn a bonus trip to the hospital gift shop if he achieved a small number of points. [see an example of a behavioral modification plan, Chap. 9, Fig. 9.1.

Nick's behavior modification plan was used to keep his initial motivation strong and start to shift patterns. Nick received a small point reward for completing his normal amount of food and then additional points for all quarter intervals above his baseline. Like many ARFID patients with sensory issues, Nick was also a selective eater. He was rewarded for trials of novel foods that the rest of the family eats. He was also rewarded for using the strategies taught by OT, including good eating posture, acupressure points, and use of an a specialized timer. Nick did not earn points for drinking the supplement since he consistently drank it within 5–10 min without difficulty.

Nick was provided with oral motor exercises that addressed chewing strength, which was weak at baseline due to delays in introducing solid foods early in life. Nick needed to more actively use his tongue to move the food from one side to the other. He practiced oral motor exercises with a nuk brush, and he was given homework to complete between sessions. During meals, OT reinforced the importance of practicing the chewing mechanics that had been taught with the nuk brushes. OT also introduced the idea of using crunchy foods to increase texture and input to the mouth between softer foods. Nick was observed to chew better when alternating crunchy textured food (i.e., chips, crunchy thinly cut carrot strips) with softer foods that gave less input (e.g., curry with rice).

As treatment progressed, OT included some exercises focusing on the amount of time spent chewing. A time timer (which counts down time in red) and an insight timer went off every 25 s to remind him to start to build a pattern of moving his food to the opposite side rather than holding it at one side all the time were utilized. OT also reinforced the importance of eating denser entree items first. Without reminders, Nick kept starting by eating his fruit and not the entrée at lunch.

Nick was discharged from the hospital and inpatient occupational therapy and was referred to outpatient occupational therapy to solidify and practice new skills with the transition home. OT encouraged the family to continue to use the behavior modification plan until the first outpatient OT session, which was in 1 month. Often behavior modification programs can help a patient transition newly learned skills from the hospital environment to their home environment and can help provide metrics for the outpatient occupational therapist regarding what the patient has done at home. After a couple of months, the behavior modification plan is typically no longer needed as the desired patterns become integrated. In Nick's case, the behavior modification plan was extended for an additional month into the outpatient treatment sessions. He continued in occupational therapy for 4 months, initially with weekly sessions, tapering to once a month in the final month. He was discharged from occupational therapy when per the medical team he continued to demonstrate weight gain and vital stability and started to diversify his nutrition with his family independent of the occupational therapist.

Chapter 15
Sensory Outpatient Case Study (Jose)

Case Presentation
Jose is a 15-year-old cisgender male with a diagnosis of Autism Spectrum Disorder (ASD) whose parents express concern about the limited food variety in his diet. Throughout childhood, Jose has been growing appropriately with a BMI that has tracked between the 50th and 75th percentiles (Fig. 15.1). His meals and snacks consist of a limited number of items including chicken nuggets (specific supermarket brand), French fries, cheese quesadillas made with Mexican cheese, and tortilla chips (specific supermarket brand). At times, he has tried different types of bread (ie, Mexican pan dulce or sweet breads) that he will eat frequently for 2–3 weeks, but then refuses secondary to being sick of it. Jose consumes a daily multivitamin. While Jose is not bothered by his food intake, his parents expressed concern that he has a 1-week long school trip that he would like to attend in 3 months. They are

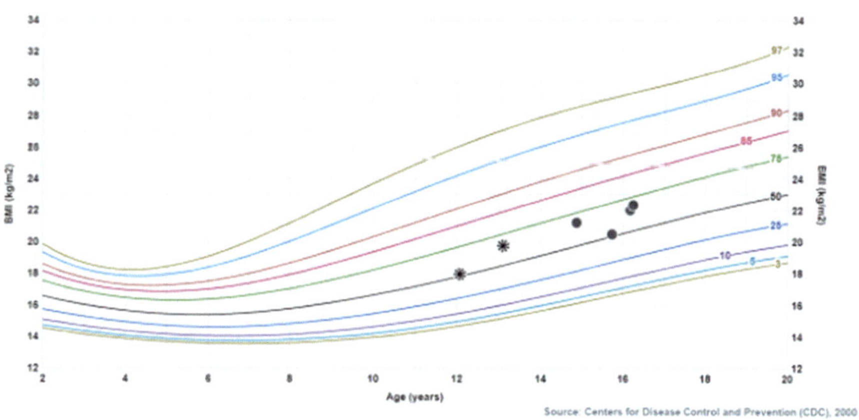

Fig. 15.1 Growth Chart for Jose

A. B. Sinha et al., *Comprehensive Clinical Care for Adolescents with Avoidant/Restrictive Food Intake Disorder (ARFID)*,
https://doi.org/10.1007/978-3-031-92232-9_15

worried that he may not be able to eat appropriately if he cannot access his preferred foods. Jose agrees that he would like to be able to join the school trip and is willing to work on increasing variety in his food repertoire. However, he isn't excited about changing his routines or preferences.

On exam, Jose appears healthy with normal vital signs.

Notable studies include: low ferritin, low 25-OH Vitamin D level.

Medical

When assessing Jose, it is notable that his limited food repertoire has not affected his growth and development. He has been able to maintain his growth trajectory, and his vital signs are currently within a normal range. This can be a typical finding in individuals whose food preferences might be limited but are not of low caloric value. Though his overall caloric intake may be appropriate, he is at risk for micronutrient deficiency due to the limited variety of food intake. Upon screening, his notable laboratory findings included a low ferritin, though not anemic, and a low 25-hydroxy Vitamin D level. To address the low ferritin, a slow-release iron supplement was recommended (every other day dosing) in addition to the inclusion of more iron-rich foods (pending the expansion of his food variety). For the low 25-OH Vitamin D level, a prescription for ergocalciferol 50,000 IU weekly for 8 weeks was initiated.

Because of his medical stability, Jose did not require intensive outpatient follow-up with the medical clinic. However, he was encouraged to follow monthly for two to three visits to ensure that he was able to maintain weight stability while focusing his efforts on an expanded food repertoire.

Psychiatry

Jose's parents were very motivated for connection to outpatient psychotherapy services focused on eating. They had been counseled in the past that he would need to be willing to engage in individual feeding therapy, and he hadn't previously been excited about doing that. Their previous experience with therapy was a group for teens with ASD that was focused on social pragmatic skills. He liked the fact that many of the participants shared his interest in Minecraft but found the activities and recommendations kind of silly. However, they all agreed that it would be a shame for him to miss out on a social experience with peers that he was looking forward to, so he said that he was willing to give it another try. With ARFID of the selective eating subtype, it is very common for the patient to have limited motivation to make change, especially if the family has been accommodating preferences long term.

Often, the desire to participate in social activities that require the ability to eat spontaneously is a very powerful motivator as the child/teen gets older.

Jose was referred to family-based treatment for ARFID (FBT-AR), and his parents were tasked with supporting him as they experimented with different ways to increase his intake variety. Previously, they would purchase preferred foods from the local store, and he would eat when hungry. He sometimes would get irritable and yell if unable to stick to his typical schedule. They took charge of planning, purchasing, preparing, and plating all meals and snacks, and implemented family meals every other evening to start. The goal of this was to ease into a meal routine that would be better for them to provide support. Jose was initially upset that this might impact his usual routine of gaming in the evening, so parents decided to eat earlier (at Jose's preferred dinner time) so they could focus on making only one change at a time. They were also able to obtain a list of commonly prepared meals/restaurants frequented on the school trip. Jose and his parents worked on reviewing the list with the therapist, and coming up with options he would be willing to try eating. They came up with a hierarchical list starting with the foods that they thought would be easiest for him to try and progressing to more challenging foods. At each session, they reviewed strategies that were helpful in allowing him to make progress, as well as those that were deemed ineffective. They learned that the process was most smooth when Jose was allowed to choose what they were working on that day. If he had a tough day at school, or wasn't feeling well, they allowed him to practice a less challenging food instead of pushing forward with something that was likely to trigger an outburst. Because he was at a normal weight and did not have any evidence of nutritional deficiencies beyond iron and vitamin D, they had the ability to be a bit more relaxed with their process.

Psychotropic medications were not indicated in this case. Jose did not have difficulty with lack of appetite, and he liked eating. He did have some generalized anxiety symptoms and mild attention deficit hyperactivity disorder, but parents preferred to focus on skills building and he seemed to do well with that. He also did not experience significant behavioral dysregulation.

Nutrition

During the initial nutrition assessment, Jose completed the 5 Food Guide.

Most of his preferred foods consisted of refined grains, fruit juices, and a variety of dessert foods. Chicken and eggs were his main protein sources. His diet had limited dairy (except for cheese), little to no fruits and vegetables, and minimal plant-based fats. When asked the #1 food he wished he could eat, Jose stated that he would like to be able to eat a burger since a lot of his classmates love to go to their local fast-food restaurant after school. His best friend (also his cousin) loves to eat the tamales that their family makes from scratch, which is another food Jose wanted to try. The dietitian agreed with those being good choices to work on, especially since those foods consist of several different foods and can have a good amount of protein.

The dietitian identified the macro- and micronutrients that were primarily missing from his diet and suggested that Jose pick out his top three foods that he's most interested in trying within the dairy, fruits, vegetables, and plant-based fats food groups. Many of the foods in the fruit and vegetable category were foods he had never heard of or seen before. The dietitian explained the food chaining process and suggested trying apples since Jose liked applesauce and mangoes since he likes mango flavored candy. Upon completion of the 5 Food Guide, the dietitian, Jose, and his family collaborated on how much to plate and what variety of food would be tried.

After obtaining a 24-h diet recall and getting an understanding of his typical meals and snacks, the dietitian created a sample meal plan for the day (Fig. 15.2) to show how Jose and his family can incorporate the newer foods into his diet. The parents were empowered to trust their instincts, and reassured that the team would work with them as they decided which strategies worked best for them.

Tuesday									
Breakfast		Lunch		Afternoon Snack		Dinner		Evening Snack	
Pan Dulce	260	Cheese pizza (1 slice)	280	5 chicken nuggets	190	Cheese quesadilla	500	Vanilla ice cream (1/2 cup)	250
Apple Juice (8 oz)	120	Potato Chips	240			Tortilla chips (1 oz)	140	Brownie (1 piece)	200
Scrambled Eggs (2) with 1 oz cheese	295	Applesauce Pouch (2)	140	Fresh apples (1 slice)		Apple juice (8 oz)	120	Milkshake (1/2 cup)	
	675		660		190		760		450
								2735	
Sunday									
Breakfast		Lunch		1400 Snack		Dinner		2000 Snack	
Pan Dulce	260	8 chicken nuggets	305	Cheetos (1 oz)	160	Cheese quesadilla (1/2)	250	Vanilla ice cream (1/2 cup)	250
Mango juice (8 oz)	120	French fries (5 oz)	215	Apple juice (8 oz)	120	French fries (3 oz)	130	Chips Ahoy cookies (3)	160
Scrambled Eggs (2) with 1 oz cheese	295	Applesauce Pouch (1)	70	Madeline cookie	140	Apple juice (8 oz)	120		
		Fresh apples (3 slices)				Fast Food Cheese-burger (1/2)	150		
	675		590		420		650		410
								2745	

Fig. 15.2 Sample meal plan for Jose

*Brand names are provided as examples only and do not imply endorsement. Selection should be based on clinical judgment and individual needs.

On Tuesday: This reflects a typical school day for Jose. To start the exposure of eating an apple, one slice was plated. Jose initially took microbites and was able to take more normal sized bites over time. While he preferred to drink apple juice or eat applesauce since it was easier to consume from an oral motor perspective, he was interested and invested in getting used to eating fresh fruit. To help increase his vitamin D level, milk was strongly encouraged but Jose wanted to consume it in a milkshake form since he hates drinking milk by itself.

On Sunday: Weekends were a better time to try more challenging, complex food exposures. The parents plated more apple slices as Jose became more successful in eating them. Jose was also able to finally try a cheeseburger and advanced from initially only taking one bite to now incorporating a half burger into his dinner meal. To accommodate this, his parents gave a smaller portion of his preferred entree food (cheese quesadilla) to help further incentivize Jose in completing the burger exposure.

The dietitian helped the family set clear expectations to help guide exposures. They decided together that newer foods had to be established ahead of time and parents agreed to follow through on providing the newer foods when first initially suggested. However, they were encouraged to trust their instincts if Jose had a challenging day and preferred to repeat a newer food instead. They set a goal of repeating newer food exposures a minimum of three times throughout the week.

To help prevent food burnout, the RD advised avoiding the same exact meal for more than two consecutive days. Instead, they agreed on rotating preferred meals and snacks, and trying different combinations of preferred foods. They were encouraged to try to introduce novel foods at the start of the meal, when Jose was most hungry, rather than at the end of the meal.

Over time, as Jose became more comfortable with eating the newer foods, the portion sizes of those foods gradually increased while the portions of his preferred foods gradually decreased to help make room for stomach volume.

Since the family decided on a behavioral modification plan to help provide positive reinforcement for the food exposures, the Eat-Replace Model was not implemented. The dietitian did mention it as an option in case Jose would find it incentivizing to keep doing exposures. Jose and his family preferred not to do replacement. While the Eat-Replace Model is often used, it was not necessary for Jose since he was of normal weight, taking a multivitamin, and eating energy dense foods. Additionally, over time, Jose was able to add newer foods to his meal plan- he gained confidence in discovering and eating new foods that he enjoyed, especially when he was able to share his eating experience with others.

Occupational Therapy

During their occupational therapy evaluation, parents reported that Jose had eaten well until the age of two, when he became more selective. He gradually eliminated previously enjoyed foods until he got to his current restricted repertoire. As noted, he had frequent food jags where he would become sick of pan dulce or tortilla chips that he previously ate regularly. Despite this, he often wanted to eat the same food repeatedly until he was tired of it.

During meal observation, he exclusively chewed on his left side, drank a lot during his meal and liked to watch videos or other media while he was eating. He seemed able to do this without it distracting from his meal, and parents agreed that this was a part of their normal home life that they did not want to change.

Occupational therapy worked with the rest of the outpatient team to get an updated list of foods that Jose had agreed to work on. A food exploration log (see Chap. 7 Fig. 7.9, Chap. 22 Appendix N) was used to track progress and gather data as Jose first experienced the newer foods. The OT talked with parents about the potential benefits of incorporating the newer foods into a reward behavior modification plan. Initially the reward was based on Jose's willingness to take three bites of the newer food at the start of the meal. A "changeover food" was consistently placed next to the newer food in case he didn't like the flavor of the newer food. When Jose reported liking a food at a rating of three or higher, they gradually worked up to having him eat between a quarter to a full portion of various items. The family set the expectation that Jose would consume the newer food first, while he still had an appetite.

Jose was alerted to his chewing patterns during OT feeding sessions and he was taught oral motor exercises (see Chap. 7 Fig. 7.8, Chap. 22 Appendix N to improve his chewing. This was especially important for the newer foods. As Jose focused on the oral motor process during eating, his insecurity about how these foods felt in his mouth started to decrease.

The family initially decided that Jose would try the newer foods in a treatment session and then they incorporated each newer food item into his dinners and weekend meal times two to three times per week to practice. Over time, his family started to spontaneously incorporate newer foods as they built the skills for introducing newer foods and incorporating them into the meal.

As time went on, the plan evolved to the following and expectations were set that once a food was consumed 20+ times a higher level of completion would be expected. Jose's parents let him know the quantity they expected which was based on a gradual increase of his baseline. Jose added several new foods and they continued to spontaneously add foods outside of treatment as they built confidence in the process. Jose tended to need more structure than peers in trying new foods (and often would only try new items initially at home) but developed confidence in his ability to taste and incorporate new food items over time.

Chapter 16
Low Interest Inpatient Case Study (Asha)

Case Presentation

Asha is a 16-year-old transgender female who was seen by her primary care provider for concerns of low appetite and weight loss. She is eating about once per day and will consume a portion of whatever dinner is being prepared by her mother. Asha denies intentional weight loss or body image concerns related to weight, though she does endorse body image issues related to gender dysphoria. Asha has been diagnosed with major depression in the past and acknowledges that her current mood is the lowest that she has experienced. She denies any interest in eating or her usual activities; she spends most of the day in bed and has been missing school.

On exam, her weight and BMI are noted to be significantly low as compared to what one would typically expect for a teenager (Fig. 16.1) She is bradycardic and orthostatic by pulse. She is referred to the inpatient medical unit for stabilization and management.

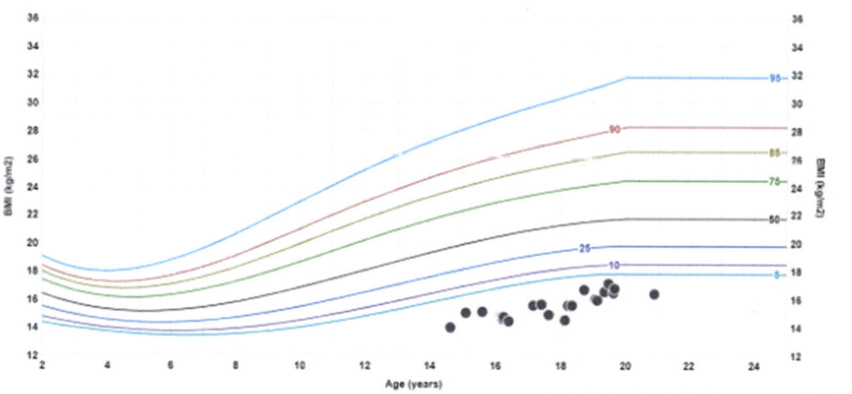

Fig. 16.1 Growth chart for Asha

A. B. Sinha et al., *Comprehensive Clinical Care for Adolescents with Avoidant/Restrictive Food Intake Disorder (ARFID)*,
https://doi.org/10.1007/978-3-031-92232-9_16

Medical

Asha was hospitalized using the inpatient admission criteria of bradycardia, orthostasis, and severe malnutrition. Based on her reported eating history (minimal) and low weight, she was also at elevated risk of refeeding syndrome and required close monitoring of her electrolytes. When her caloric intake began to improve, she was noted to have drops below the normal range in her phosphorus levels, and she required oral phosphorus supplementation for stabilization. Prior to discharge, her phosphorus supplementation was able to be weaned off. Demonstration of normal phosphorus levels without supplementation is a typical goal for discharge.

To improve Asha's vital signs, it was critical to improve her nutritional status. However, due to her underlying depression and expected delay in response to SSRIs, Asha struggled with the eat- and replace model that is typically utilized for low-interest ARFID. Using shared decision making, it was decided to place a nasogastric tube to implement the eat-replace model until Asha was motivated to complete the replacement by mouth. Any nutrition that she could not take by mouth would be administered after the mealtime via bolus nasogastric tube feeds. Once she was able to do all her prescribed nutrition by mouth for two meals/snacks in a row, the nasogastric tube could be removed, and the typical eat and replace model would continue. Within her first week of admission, Asha was able to transition to all oral nutrition and have her tube removed without need for subsequent replacement.

Psychiatry

During Asha's evaluation, she underscored a long history of gender dysphoria which seemed to drive her depression. She also experienced long term indifference to food at baseline, although she hadn't previously had such a significant decrease in appetite. Diminished interest and appetite had been associated with low mood for several years now, although she also notes that being thin does seem to help her feel a little more confident in her body. Despite major depressive disorder being primary, the diagnosis of ARFID was also made, given that the weight loss had become significant enough that Asha needed to be medically hospitalized for malnutrition secondary to low appetite/low interest which required specialty eating disorder treatment.

The primary focus for the psychiatry team was to target the symptoms of depression. They worked with Asha on cognitive behavioral therapy (CBT) techniques including helping her adhere to a structure that encouraged her to be out of bed and interacting with people during the daytime hours. She also made sure to prioritize hygiene and other acts of self-care. With the assistance of her therapist, she practiced identifying and restructuring distorted thoughts, added daily pleasurable activities to her schedule, and began to cultivate a mindfulness and gratitude practice. She also identified life goals that she was looking forward to achieving.

Asha agreed to a trial of fluoxetine, which was initiated at low dose and did seem to help energize her a bit. The psychiatrist worked with the medical team to review the admission EKG and labs to be sure that Asha wasn't experiencing any issues with prolonged QTc, which is sometimes an issue in severe malnutrition. It is also important to note that the team talked with Asha and her family at length about the limitations of antidepressants when someone is inadequately nourished. The SSRIs do not work optimally in malnutrition, so renourishment remains the most important intervention. As Asha was able to take in consistent nutrition and engage in stimulating activities, her mood began to improve, and she noticed that her hunger and fullness cues started to return.

Nutrition

With the RD, Asha described her typical school day and weekend day, and what she ate. On school days, she struggled to wake up in the morning and typically got ready for school at the very last minute, often fixing her hair or putting on makeup in the car. She rarely ate breakfast and mostly sipped on a chai tea latte. During lunch period, she would read or spend time with her best friend. She denied being ravenous at this time, despite not eating breakfast, and said she would typically feel satiated after eating a bag of chips, some apple slices, and a beverage like iced tea. After school, she would stop by the convenience store and get a candy bar if she was hungry. Asha knew her mom would nag her about eating so she usually ate the most during dinner time. The rest of the evening she spent time in her room.

Weekends consisted of a similar intake, although she suspects that she ate less since she mostly spent time in bed and disliked a lot of the snacks at home since they were "too healthy" or "boring" like nuts or dried fruit. Considering Asha's minimal intake prior to admission, especially during the day, the RD modified her breakfast and lunch meals to be smaller, almost the size of snacks, and made the dinner meal the biggest meal of the day. To help meet her calorie goals, breakfast and lunch included energy dense foods such as fried foods, whole milk dairy items, baked goods, and desserts. Although Asha didn't mind eating the hospital food, she would get too full, bored, or tired to eat after 10–15 min and elected to do NGT replacement to complete the remainder of her nutrition during the first week of her admission. Eventually she was able to eat most of her meals and snacks with some oral replacement needed. Her replacement was also changed to a denser formula since Asha had early satiety and struggled if the replacement volume was too high.

Using the 5 Food Guide, the RD collaborated with Asha and created a sample meal plan for 1 week. The RD emphasized the importance of following a consistent meal and snack schedule and reminded Asha that she cannot fully rely on her hunger and fullness cues at this time. Instead, Asha would need to rely on a specified plan and schedule to help meet her nutrition needs. Asha anticipated that she would "get lazy" with her meal plan and she worried about how easy it would be to not keep eating so the RD included a lot of easy to grab foods, pre-portioned items, convenient meals and snacks, and shelf-stable foods to keep in her room or backpack.

Over time, the RD recommended that Asha work with her outpatient team to consider having an end of the day replacement plan rather than eat-or-replace at every meal or snack since that approach can require more effort by the patient and/or family.

Occupational Therapy

When meeting with occupational therapy, Asha presented with a flat affect. She had trouble defining her goals of treatment. She reported an 8/10 desire to get better and a 6/10 desire to work at it, a discrepancy that was noted by the OT. Asha's primary barriers to eating were feeling tired, not feeling hungry and getting full easily. Asha reported that although she thought she had liked food in the past, lately she felt she fit in the "eat to live" category as opposed to "live to eat". Asha was taught an acupressure point for early satiety (Fig. 7.2) prior to the first meal session.

OT met privately with Asha's mom. She reported keeping the pantry and fridge well-stocked with many foods that she has seen Asha eat, but notes that Asha never eats them unless mom warms them and hands them to her. Her mother expressed concern about whether Asha would be able to remember to stop to eat regularly when she goes to college in a couple years. Asha's mom agreed to order a high calorie shake powder to mix with 8 oz milk for use at home post-discharge, as well as expressed support for reinforcing OT taught strategies.

Asha had a typical chewing pattern but prolonged mealtimes. She tended to take sips of her water regularly and indicated that she enjoyed beverages like milk and juice. During mealtime, Asha was observed to put both of her knees against her chest. When asked why, she reported that she found this position comforting.

Based on the initial observations, it was decided that Asha was allowed the typical amount of time (30 min at breakfast and snacks, 40 min at lunch and dinner) to complete meals and snacks, but was given an extra 15 min at dinner. Replacement was provided in the final 10 min of the meal or snacks. Lunch was adjusted so that she had more time before the next snack (feeling full was from lunch often a barrier to eating in the afternoon). It was noted that she could have optional food items or foods she could trade out (from her family/ outside or readily available food on the unit) to encourage her to eat as much as possible. Calorie containing beverages were added to her tray to optimize calorie intake while eating and she was encouraged to keep her feet on the ground and sit upright during mealtimes.

To help Asha develop some insight and ownership into her physical need for nutrition, OT provided education about how regular fuel has an influence on cognition, focus, mood, and physical health. Asha's mom shared concerns about sending her away to college in the future if she isn't eating enough to support her health and wellbeing, so they discussed how to increase her level of responsibility and how to make eating an expected activity of daily living like brushing her teeth or doing homework. OT worked with the family to develop structure including a daily ADL routine (brushing teeth and hair, showering) and attending all groups while hospitalized to reinforce routines that would help her return to school while building up her endurance for daytime activity.

At discharge, Asha was referred to outpatient occupational therapy to help her transition her new routines to her home environment and continue to skill build around participation in her daily ADLs and getting adequate nutrition at regular intervals.

Chapter 17
Low Interest Outpatient Case Study (Adam)

Case Presentation

Adam is a 16-year-old cisgender male with attention deficit hyperactivity disorder (ADHD) who presents for concern of low weight. His parents remark that he has never seemed interested in food and has always needed encouragement and reminders to eat enough. He consumes a variety of foods and is not considered "picky" by his family. Adam denies any body image concerns and remarks that he would like to be of a normal weight. He states that he doesn't feel hungry and tends to become full easily.

Adam takes methylphenidate-extended release (ER) for his ADHD with good success. Without his medication, parents report that he gets in a lot of trouble at school for talking and distracting the class. He has trouble waking up in the morning to eat an adequate breakfast before leaving for school. At lunch, he reports that he isn't hungry, and prefers to spend the time allocated for lunch playing basketball with his friends instead. Once he is home, his parents notice that he is a little hungrier as his stimulant medicine wears off, but they have a difficult time getting him to attend to eating due to problems with distractibility and his preference for playing video games.

On exam, Adam has not lost any weight, but his weight percentile is trending lower than in the past (Fig. 17.1). His vital signs are stable.

Notable studies include: low 25-OH Vitamin D.

A. B. Sinha et al., *Comprehensive Clinical Care for Adolescents with Avoidant/Restrictive Food Intake Disorder (ARFID)*,
https://doi.org/10.1007/978-3-031-92232-9_17

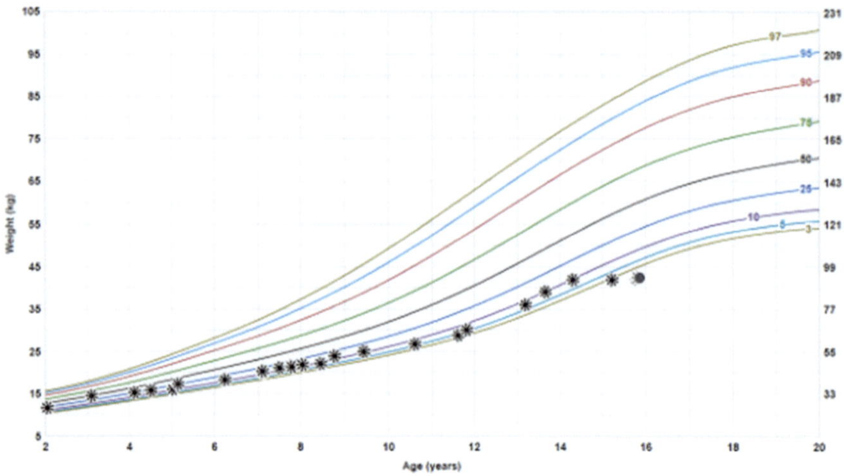

Fig. 17.1 Growth Chart for Adam

Medical

Though Adam had not lost any weight, his weight percentiles declined because he was not able to make the weight gain expected for his age. This discrepancy can be particularly notable during adolescence when individuals are expected to gain significant amounts of weight and height. Adam's medical evaluation did not reveal other etiologies to explain his lack of weight progress. Reassuringly, his vital signs were normal. His blood work was notable for low Vitamin D, a typical sequela of malnutrition. This was repleted with ergocaciferol 50,000 international units weekly for 8 weeks.

As Adam was medically stable and able to engage with therapy, OT, and nutrition, he did not require a high level of medical intervention or supervision. He was medically followed at 4-to-6-week intervals to ensure that he was making weight progress. After several consecutive visits in which he demonstrated a positive weight trend, he was discharged from the outpatient eating disorder medical clinic.

Psychiatry

Adam was engaged with his therapist, and they primarily worked on executive coaching strategies to keep himself organized at school. For example, he was able to get an accommodation such that he was able to take a photo of the homework agenda that the teacher sets for each class. He also made sure to set alarms and reminders to turn his homework in on time. He had flexible deadlines, but tried hard to follow a schedule so that he stayed on top of his study schedule.

Adam's parents had previously been told that they needed to stop the methylphenidate ER (concerta) because of growth concerns, but his function decreased dramatically when they did so. In addition to worsening grades, he had trouble staying on top of his activities of daily living, and his room was a "disaster zone." They also tried other stimulant medications, but all of them decreased his appetite. His mother commented that he seemed to have more trouble eating when he was off medication because he was so distracted and had difficulty attending to his meal.

Adam's psychiatrist agreed that treating the ADHD was likely an important part of helping him get enough nutrition. He created a contract with Adam, whereby he would continue to write prescriptions for medications if Adam made progress with weight gain. In the beginning, they dropped by the office for observed weights and vital signs each week, and the psychiatrist filled the prescription after making sure everything looked stable. They struggled a bit with adherence to requested visits, and Adam was not always consistent with taking his medication as recommended. Over time, after they had built trust, they decreased the cadence of visits until they were able to have parents get a supervised weight at home, which they sent to the psychiatrist monthly. Adam had a few weigh-ins where he had lost a few pounds, and the psychiatrist stayed true to the contract and held the medication. Adam was upset, and parents tried to get the psychiatrist to change his mind, but they soon recognized that Adam functioned better on his medication, and needed it to be able to achieve the things that were important to him. This knowledge helped everyone be more consistent with the plan. Adam asked his therapist if they could work on adding a plan to increase structure and create a nutrition back-up to be sure he wasn't tempted to skip meals when he was distracted or just not hungry. They also experimented with his wake-up time, so that he could get in a robust breakfast before his medication fully kicked in, and he carried nutrient dense snacks in his backpack, so he always had access to a meal, even when running late.

Nutrition

During the first outpatient session, RD emphasized the importance of following a set meal/snack schedule to provide consistency and follow through with nutrition. Together, they created a schedule that was realistic to follow every day of the week that included three meals and two snacks per day. Alarms were set on his phone to specify the start time of each eating interval. Parents were advised to set time limits around meals: 30 minutes for meals and 15 min for snacks. A plan was set such that Adam was allowed to be excused to play video games if he was able to finish 100% of the food before time ends. If he was unable to finish 100% of the food, then the meal/snack time would be extended by 10 extra minutes so he can finish replacement instead. Missed nutrition was replaced by a liquid supplement. Every meal was equivalent to 2 bottles of a High-calorie, nutritionally complete oral supplement (~1.5 kcal/mL) and every snack was equivalent to 1 bottle of the supplement. The family appreciated the idea of implementing structure and Adam appreciated the simplicity of the replacement plan.

Although Adam expressed wanting to gain weight and understood the importance of nutrition, his actions were often incongruent with his goal. Parents reported that Adam struggled to come to the table as he often was in the middle of something and would delay the start time. Consequently, meals and snacks would be off schedule and the family struggled to get back on track. On some days, Adam heavily relied on replacement "just to get it over with" which also frustrated parents as they strongly desired for him to eat the food. Adam shared that he worried that he might try to eat the food, not finish, and still need replacement anyways. Therefore, he felt like it would just be easier to just drink the replacement, especially on busy days. RD commended Adam for vulnerably sharing his thoughts and explained that nourishment from actual food is going to be an ongoing nutrition goal since (1) his body benefits from digestion and absorption of nutrients from food, (2) to prevent burnout from nutritional supplements, (3) and to keep eating a variety of foods to obtain a variety of essential nutrients.

The RD worked with the family to brainstorm food items that are dense and easy-to-consume to help keep Adam interested in eating. It was a motivator for Adam to finish a meal early so he could get back to doing his preferred activities. RD recommended breakfast sandwiches, adding a smoothie or milkshake to lunches at school, or pairing nuts with a smoothie for an after-school snack. She encouraged parents to cook more dense entrees such as shepherd's pie, lasagna, or pasta for dinner and suggested ice cream or dessert items for evening snack since they are easy to eat. Adam disliked drinking milk by itself and refused to finish his milk when eating it with cereal. The RD advised including more milk in smoothies or milkshakes to help address his low Vitamin D status. The RD provided a sample meal plan to help Adam and his family visualize how much food is needed to help meet his nutritional needs. The Ladder Block Plan also helped Adam stay on track with his meal/snack schedule as well as his nutritional needs. Over time, he was able to consume adequate calories, and exhibit appropriate weight gain.

During ongoing sessions, the RD advised parents to always provide a preferred food at meals to help stimulate his appetite and bring his attention back to the meal. She encouraged Adam to drink water in between meals so it does not compete with stomach volume at mealtime. She also encouraged starting occupational therapy.

Occupational Therapy

Adam was referred by his adolescent medicine doctor to rule out any oral motor difficulties and to help support Adam in a consistent eating schedule. He had already started working with the psychiatrist and the RD when occupational therapy was initiated.

In evaluation, it was found that Adam frequently overslept, skipped meals and tended to chew on one side. Additional education about the impact of nutrition on the mind, body and focus was provided. Adam was taught oral motor exercises and had meals with the OT to address his chewing pattern. He was encouraged to add crunchy food between bites when he felt distracted or bored by chewing. Over time he showed improvement in his chewing pattern and efficiency while eating. While this did not change his interest in eating, (he still felt he had better things to do) it did make it easier.

The potential use of the Ladder Block Plan was discussed with his parents as a reinforcer of food quantity and timeliness, and they felt it would give them and Adam a concrete way to know if he was getting enough food and help him stay on track. They reported that he responds well to rewards and asked that a reward component be added. After brainstorming it was found that Adam often asked for money to spend on small things while gaming but parents rarely provided it. It was decided that he could earn some money that would be added to his gaming portal (up to \$5–10/ week depending on how he did). Adam was thrilled with this as a reward and found it motivating. Adam and his parents felt that the use of the Ladder Block Plan (see Chap. 8) helped all of them have a clearer idea of how to keep up with this nutrition and also helped them see how tough it was to catch up if he got behind. After a while, use of the block plan became very natural, and the family decided they did not need it anymore. They were reassured to know that they could always resurrect it if he went through a transition (like a new job) or was struggling, and they were proud that the skills had been incorporated. Adam's parents would still remind him to complete his blocks if Adam seemed disinterested or unfocused while eating. At that point, parents decided to shift his behavior modification rewards towards keeping his room clean and doing some household chores. He was discharged from OT after eight outpatient sessions spread over 4 months, with more frequent sessions initially and less frequent sessions as his nutrition and routine stabilized.

Chapter 18
Fear of Aversive Consequences Inpatient Case Study (Sally)

Case Presentation
Sally is a 11.5 year old cisgender female who reports generalized anxiety, including fear of choking for the past several years. Her anxiety has worsened in the past 6 months, and she has been on the waitlist for a medication evaluation with Psychiatry for the past 3 months. About 6 weeks ago, she witnessed a friend choke while eating a hot dog. Following that episode, her parents noted that she appeared anxious around food and started having progressively worsening vomiting episodes around mealtime. They are divorced, but communicate frequently. Sally began to increasingly restrict her intake to the point of consuming only a few sips of milk or juice. She denies any body image concerns or weight loss goals.

Three weeks ago, she presented to her PCP due to her minimal food intake and vomiting. She was started on cyprohepatidine with the hopes of improving her overall appetite. During her follow-up visit 3 weeks later, her intake continued to be minimal and she was now reporting fatigue and dizziness. She was noted to be bradycardic and hypotensive on vital sign measurement and was referred to the inpatient medical unit for stabilization and management.

Medical

Sally's bradycardia, prolonged QTc, hypotension, and severe malnutrition meet medical admission criteria. Her inpatient medical stability consisted of minimizing her activity, improving her nutritional intake, and monitoring for refeeding syndrome. Given her minimal nutritional intake and low weight, Sally was at very high risk for refeeding syndrome. Her vomiting could also exacerbate hypokalemia that might occur with refeeding. Her laboratory values were monitored daily for the first week of her admission. She did require oral supplementation with phosphorus for 5

A. B. Sinha et al., *Comprehensive Clinical Care for Adolescents with Avoidant/Restrictive Food Intake Disorder (ARFID)*,
https://doi.org/10.1007/978-3-031-92232-9_18

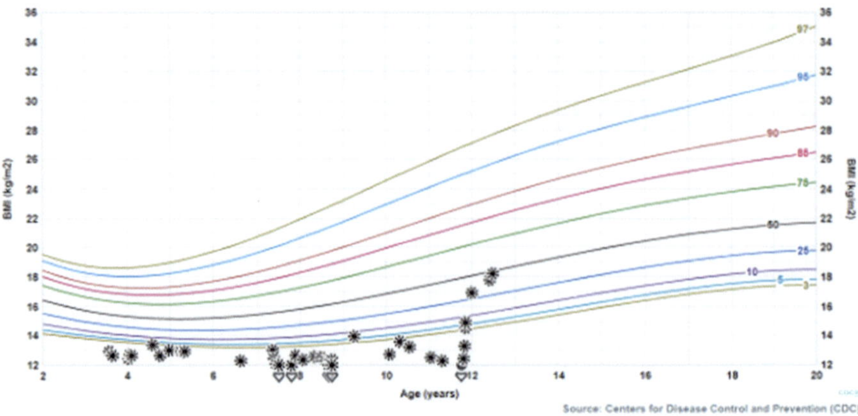

Fig. 18.1 Growth chart for Sally

days; her dosing was titrated to ensure that her levels remained on the higher side of the normal value range. Prior to discharge, her phosphorus was able to be weaned completely.

During her admission, the use of cyproheptadine was discussed. Sally had not found it to be helpful for appetite stimulation, and it is not frequently useful in patients with the fear of aversive consequences subtype of ARFID. In addition, cyproheptadine has anti-serotinergic properties that can interfere with any SSRI medications being initiated. Due to these factors, it was decided to discontinue cyproheptadine.

As Sally worked with the team members during her admission, her weight improved, and her vital signs stabilized. Her symptoms of dizziness and fatigue resolved, and she was able to manage her abdominal fullness. She did have issues with constipation which is not uncommon when patients are increasing their intake while remaining restful. For constipation, she was prescribed polyethylene glycol to effectively manage her symptoms. She was discharged with plans to continue to follow-up in the outpatient clinics where she continued to make progress (Fig. 18.1).

Notable studies include an EKG with heart rate of 41 and QTc of 485 ms.

Psychiatry

Evaluation with child psychiatry on the inpatient service confirmed a longstanding history of anxiety in all settings, with a pattern of "jumping" from one area of preoccupation to another. She and her parents note that she has had lifelong fears, intrusive worry thoughts, and physical sensations of jitteriness and feeling on edge. Currently, she seems completely preoccupied with worries about choking and vomiting, whereas prior to the event, she was mostly convinced that an intruder was trying to break into their home through her bedroom window. Given how life impairing her symptoms have been, the family has been amenable to a trial of an SSRI or other medication to help mitigate her baseline symptoms.

Sally was significantly impacted by witnessing her friend choking on a hot dog. Thankfully, her friend was able to clear the hot dog on her own with vigorous coughing and did not require any additional medical intervention. Sally remains plagued by re-experiencing the event and avoids the cafeteria where this happened. She feels nervous and on edge, and now has a sensation in her own throat while eating that makes her worry that she might choke when eating various foods. While she used to eat small portions of all foods, she has begun to narrow her dietary repertoire, noticing that she has a lump in her throat while eating certain foods. She is nervous before every meal and snack. She meets criteria for ARFID, while also experiencing symptoms consistent with an acute stress reaction that could potentially evolve into Post Traumatic Stress Disorder (PTSD). Technically the DSM says that you should not make an ARFID diagnosis in someone where the symptoms are better explained by another condition, but in this case, it is warranted given the need for specialty eating disorder care.

Given that the family has been on board with the idea of an SSRI, it was recommended that she start a low dose of sertraline once her QTc showed signs of improvement. The EKG can normalize with renourishment, but it is important to monitor, and make sure that magnesium and potassium levels are optimized to reduce the risk of torsades des pointes. The team consulted with cardiology, who agreed with starting a medication once the QTc was closer to 450 ms, monitoring the EKG, and minimizing use of other agents that could potentially prolong the QTc (such as ondansetron that is sometimes prescribed to combat nausea in the ARFID population).

Nutrition

During the initial nutrition assessment, Sally shared that her primary food sources were whole milk, chocolate milk, white grape juice, apple juice, and chocolate Pediasure (mixed with chocolate syrup). She had been able to tolerate some other foods such as yogurt, finely mashed avocados, rice, and soup but severely limited her intake to just liquids after constantly vomiting at almost every meal and snack. Although Sally was started on the standard meal plan with an "eat and replace" model, she quickly was changed to an "ad lib" meal plan where the family could bring outside foods to help meet her nutrition needs. Seeing more familiar foods and beverages helped decrease Sally's anxiety around eating, which in turn, helped her better tolerate the meals and snacks. As Sally learned how to avoid vomiting, her solid foods expanded. Sally was provided three meals and two snacks per day. The RD collaborated closely with the OT to encourage specific foods and textures at mealtimes in order to work on improving her chewing pattern.

Below are samples of specific combo of foods to help practice chewing pattern while fostering efficiency with completion:

- Mac and cheese and thinly cut carrots.
- Banana bread with apple slices
- Pretzels with hummus, guacamole with hummus
- Chips and cheese

Prescribing a certain amount of Pediasure at every meal and snack for a period of time helped provide ~500 calories per day. To help expedite weight repletion, Sally was introduced to higher calorie formulas, Boost Kids Essentials 1.5 and Pediasure 1.5.

As Sally completed food exposures, gained weight, and developed confidence with eating solids, she was able to progress and meet her nutrition needs primarily through solid foods. The RD discovered that food chaining with soft foods was only needed very briefly, and Sally rapidly returned to eating her previously preferred foods. The family felt confident that they didn't need a detailed meal plan on discharge. Instead, they knew the amount of food she needed at meals and snacks and understood that Pediasure could be used to fully meet her needs when she struggled with completing her nutrition (Fig. 18.2).

Sally's meal plan upon hospital discharge included some foods from home (Fig. 18.2). She was able to have a mix of soft and solid food items and no longer needed a prescribed amount of formula to drink at every meal and snack. This meal plan shows how much food is needed at her estimated calorie goal of 2500 kcal/day.

DAY 8		2500 KCAL							
Breakfast		Lunch		1400 Snack		Dinner		2000 Snack	
Strawberry Yogurt (6 oz)	140	FROM HOME: Kids Subway Sandwich - Black Forest Ham	170	Vanilla Milkshake (8 oz)	305	Chicken Tenders (3 pcs)	300	Vanilla Ice Cream Cup (1/2 cup)	130
FROM HOME: Blueberry Muffin	460	Cranberry Juice (4 oz)	60	Fresh Strawberries (1 cup)	50	French Fries (3 oz)	275	FROM HOME: Tate's Cookies (choc chip) (2)	140
Whole Milk (8 oz)	160	Potato Chips (1 oz)	150			Apple Juice (8 oz)	120	Water	
		Mixed Fresh Fruit (1 cup)	70						
	760		450		355		695		270
								2530	

Fig. 18.2 Sample meal plan for Sally

Occupational Therapy

Sally's reported barriers to typical eating included: nausea, fear of nausea, emesis, fear of vomiting, stomach pain, feeling too full and fear of choking. Prior to her first mealtime session, Sally was taught strategies to avoid vomiting (e.g., abdominal breathing with loose body posture to avoid emesis). She was also taught how to know if she was choking (See Chap. 7, Video 7.10), and what to do if she did choke. She was taught pressure points for nausea and fullness and was provided with a Reliefband trial for addressing nausea.

At the first mealtime session, it was also observed that Sally demonstrated immature oral motor patterns (per family these were lifelong) and delayed swallow patterns (related to fear of choking) significantly impacting her ability to achieve adequate nutritional intake. After the first occupational therapy feeding session the initial eat and replace plan was paused, and Sally was transitioned to an "ad lib" diet and was allowed to trade foods from home as desired (with team approval).

The team also recommended trying to avoid fluid for 30 min before and 60 min after meals and to take small sips if needed with meals to help prevent excess fluid that can increase the likelihood of vomiting (see Chap. 7, Video 7.9 and order references in Feeding Plan Chap. 22). Of note, for patients who vomit two or more times per day, fluids are often completely separated from meals. However, Sally drank extensively while eating due to a fear of choking and to provide sensory input to her throat in an attempt to keep it clear. As a result, fluids were reduced rather than completely removed.

Sally was provided a twice per day oral motor exercise program to address her chewing pattern, and received extensive education about a typical swallow pattern, which she practiced with water outside of mealtimes. She was also provided with Theraputty as a potential fidget distractor as she tended to move a lot during sessions. Starburst candies were introduced as a motivator, reward, and strategy for increasing calories as well as improving chewing mechanics and strength.

With the support of her family, the Ladder Block Plan was initiated on hospital day five. Sally's overall intake had increased enough to be reliable, she had been able to achieve 2 oz. of supplement at breakfast through dinner and she had not vomited for over 24 h. Nursing provided training in family meals (training parents individually in the use of the ladder block plan and in the FBT model of support during meals). Nursing provided an ARFID family training hand-out prior to starting the first family meal. Since Sally had achieved the ability to take the 2 oz. of supplement (and could perceive it as a mealtime supplement) this was no longer required with meals and snacks. Instead, with the Ladder Block Plan, the patient understood that she could meet her nutritional blocks through any means. This included food presented on her tray, food that her family added, food readily available on the unit (i.e, easy access refrigerated food such as yogurt, crackers, cheese sticks, drinks), dry food kept on the unit (i.e., crackers, peanut butter, etc.) or through an oral supplement. Sally's Ladder Block Plan included a behavioral incentive point component that had been collaboratively developed with the family. Parents brainstormed a list of special outings that they were committed to providing as a reward for earning points as part of the Ladder Block Plan. It was important to choose activities that were outside the range of typical family activities. When it became clear that Sally seemed to struggle to complete her blocks more with one parent than the other (e.g. more commonly used the supplementation with one parent), the team worked to help the parents work together to develop consistent strategies to be consistent and to provide gentle support, in a neutral and non-judgmental manner. Blocks gradually progressed to the goal of 2470 kcals.

Sally did have an episode of emesis after eating a hamburger. OT worked with her to repeat the same food the next day to make sure that she did not avoid and inadvertently reinforce the anxiety. She was able to eat 20% of it and make her blocks at that meal through a combination of food and supplement without emesis. Sally also reported constipation and her progress slowed. The medical team started medicine and recommended increasing fluids. The occupational therapist provided additional education, created a fluid log (see sample in Chap. 22, Appendix I), and instructed her in the use of a footstool and muscle coordination coaching to optimize voiding (see Chap. 22, Appendix D).

Even at discharge, Sally continued to require extensive cues about her chewing and swallowing pattern, though family members reported that her chewing had improved. She was referred to an outpatient occupational therapist who specialized in ARFID to work on transitioning to using the skills she was taught to her in the hospital to her home environment and to continue to address oral motor skills. At Sally's initial outpatient adolescent medicine and RD follow-up, she had lost weight, but at the subsequent follow-ups, she restored weight each time and continued to make progress until she was back to her baseline eating patterns and developed improvement in her oral motor patterns.

Chapter 19
Fear of Aversive Consequences Inpatient Case Study (Tim)

Case Presentation

Tim is an 18-year-old cisgender male with a history of generalized anxiety and previously diagnosed ARFID (sensory subtype). He had been doing well with his nutritional intake until experiencing an episode of viral gastroenteritis that resulted in vomiting and weight loss (Fig. 19.1). Upon recovery from the viral syndrome, Tim was not able to increase his intake, as expected, due to continued worry about vomiting. When seen by his PCP, he was found to be bradycardic (heart rate of 35 beats per minute) and had profound weight loss. He was referred to the inpatient medical unit for stabilization and management.

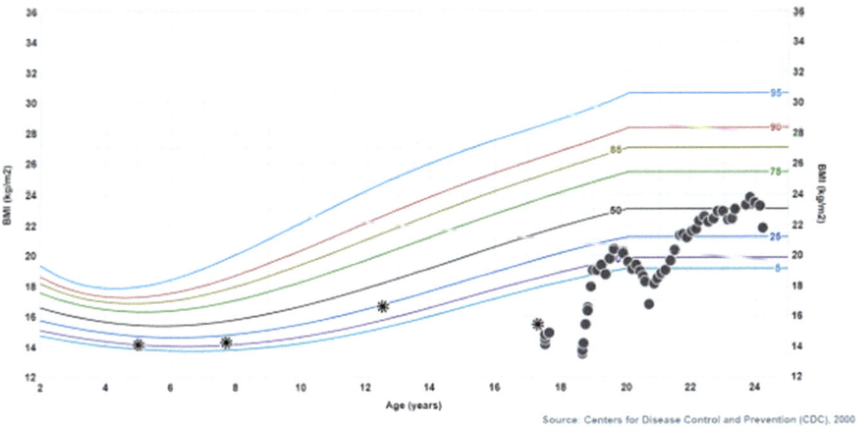

Fig. 19.1 Growth chart for Tim

A. B. Sinha et al., *Comprehensive Clinical Care for Adolescents with Avoidant/Restrictive Food Intake Disorder (ARFID)*,
https://doi.org/10.1007/978-3-031-92232-9_19

Upon admission to the medical unit, Tim stated that he wanted to improve his weight and stabilize his vital signs. However, he worried that he would not be able to take more than a few bites or sips of nutrition. He asked if he could be fed with a tube (Fig. 19.1).

Medical

At the time of admission, Tim met the medical admission criteria of profound bradycardia (heart rate of 35) and severe malnutrition (BMI less than 75% of median BMI for age). Given the level of his bradycardia, he needed to be initiated on an appropriate nutritional plan immediately. His request to use a nasogastric tube for nutrition was discussed and determined to be the most medically appropriate modality for effectively delivering his nutrition. He was started on

nasogastric feeding at a continuous rate for 24 h/day. The continuous feeding plan was chosen to minimize gastric distress/vomiting potential while ensuring an appropriate amount of nutrition being delivered. Once team members worked on coping skills for nausea and vomiting, Tim felt comfortable to switch the feeling plan to overnight nasogastric feeding with opportunities to consume food items by mouth throughout the day. As he medically stabilized, the amount of nighttime feeding was decreased, and the daytime oral intake was increased until he reached a point of being able to discontinue the supplemental tube feeding altogether.

As Tim presented at a low weight with minimal nutritional intake, he was at elevated risk of refeeding syndrome. This risk was further complicated by his need for higher levels of nutrition to improve his very low heart rate. His electrolytes were monitored daily for the first week of his admission. He did require oral phosphorus supplementation which was able to be weaned prior to discharge.

Tim was discharged with stable vital signs, improved weight, and ability to consume his nutrition by mouth. His follow-up plan included weekly medical follow-up to monitor his outpatient progress.

Psychiatry

Tim was incredibly insightful about his eating difficulties and had previously used an NG tube to supplement his intake when he was struggling with his nutrition. In the past, the issue was primarily related to challenges expanding his food repertoire. More recently, he was able to tolerate a wider range of foods but struggled with fear of vomiting after his viral illness.

Tim and his hospital therapist began working on CBT techniques, and they were able to identify and challenge his fear that he would get sick if he ate more. They developed a list of coping strategies and techniques to distract himself when anxious. While he was on NG tube feeds, he did imaginary exposures to start to build confidence and practice using those skills. When he was medically ready to start eating solid food again, he participated in meal exposures. Between sessions, he agreed to complete homework at meals and snacks where he challenged himself to do the things he feared most. For example, he committed to having another two bites past the point when he began to worry that he was going to vomit. He also made a goal to become comfortable with eating chicken soup again. He had been trying to eat it to soothe his stomach when he was ill, but now associated it with vomiting.

Tim also agreed to resume his psychiatric medications. He had been on a small dose of mirtazapine to help increase his appetite and interest in food but stopped it when he no longer felt that it was needed. With the weight loss, he noticed a relapse into a higher anxiety state. The mirtazapine decreased the nausea he experienced and allowed him to fall asleep with fewer anxious ruminations about vomiting.

Occupational Therapy and Nutrition

When occupational therapy assessed Tim, he reported a 10/10 desire to get better and a 7/10 willingness to work at it "because I feel afraid." His biggest barriers to eating were fear of vomiting and nausea. He explained that he had two types of nausea: over-hunger and anxiety. Tim felt hungry all the time and was not feeling over-full but could only take bites of food despite being able to eat an entire applesauce cup. He reported feeling certain that an NG tube would help him as he reported feeling much weaker than usual and was worried that "getting better will take forever."

At the initial occupational therapy eval, Tim was taught strategies for avoiding vomiting and tried a Reliefband to address nausea. Tim did not like the vibration feeling in his wrist and instead preferred Acubands and lavender aromatherapy. Initially, he struggled with abdominal breathing with relaxed body posture, and had to practice it while lying down for several days before he was able to transition to abdominal breathing in a seated position. He was also observed to tighten his shoulders while speaking about anxiety provoking topics but responded well to verbal cues and repeated practice to build relaxation skills.

The RD collaborated with Tim on his nutrition plan, and they decided to start NG tube feeds as his main nutrition source for the initial 2 days. While Tim was continuously nourished via the tube, he planned to actively work on skills to combat nausea and vomiting. He felt that the tube feeds provided temporary relief and a break from worry thoughts related to eating. Considering Tim was volume restricted, the most energy dense formula was chosen for his feeds. He tolerated the initiation well, and the rate was increased gradually to goal.

After 2 days of continuous NGT feeds, he transitioned to overnight feeds from 10 p.m. to 6 a.m. and was encouraged to increase his daytime PO intake. Breakfast was not provided since most of his nutritional intake occurred overnight and ended at 6 a.m. Tim was understandably not hungry in the mornings and needed to gradually stimulate his appetite by early afternoon. With the team's collaboration, Tim worked on planned food exposures from morning snack at 10 am to evening snack at 8 pm.

At every meal and snack, applesauce was provided on the tray since that was Tim's safe food. Using his completed 5 Food Guide, the RD provided an array of previously enjoyed foods as well, with an emphasis on aromatic foods (such as a burger and French fries, chicken tenders, and chocolate cake) to help stimulate his olfactory senses and appetite.

As anticipated, Tim only took a few bites of food at his initial exposure session. Tim agreed that a behavior modification plan (without formal rewards) would help positively reinforce his participation in working on bites of food and use of productive coping strategies. Expectations were gradually increased from bites, to consuming a fourth and then one half of the serving presented. Once he was more consistently completing solid food, replacement was introduced as a strategy to increase his oral intake. Tim taste-tested various supplements in session, ultimately choosing a vanilla high calorie oral supplement. He was able to gradually increase the volume of supplement consumed. Along the way, input from Tim and from his family was essential in helping craft a plan with the highest chances of long-term success. For example, they gave feedback on the timing of the meals and snacks and determined that adding something salty (like chips) helped him better tolerate the sweet flavor of the supplement. Using these methods, the team was able to decrease overnight feeds and increase the number of calories consumed orally during the day.

After demonstrating a consistent PO intake of 1000 kcal, which included supplement at every meal and snack, for 48 h, the team implemented the Ladder Block Plan (see Chaps. 8, 12). This plan provided a visual of the blocks of nutrition he was getting at each meal and snack (colored in green) and the overnight nutrition (colored in gray). The team shared that the goal was to step-by-step move from having the nutrition overnight to incorporating it into the day. Tim endorsed that he was starting to feel physically stronger from receiving more nutrition and mentally stronger as he experienced increased mastery over the things that caused him significant anxiety.

For the Ladder Block Plan, there were 8 total blocks with each block value set at 200 calories. Initially all the block values except for morning and evening snacks were set at equal intervals of 2 blocks. Tim could choose whether he wanted some supplement as a method of making his blocks. It was also offered when he felt unable to consume more food. Tim's NGT feeds were gradually weaned. Breakfast was then offered and a block for this was added to his Ladder Block Plan.

Over time, the night feeds decreased until only 400 kcals remained. At that point the feed was fully weaned and an additional block was added to the evening snack so that Tim was consuming 2400 day time calories PO.

The NG was kept as a back-up as Tim had a lot of anxiety about his ability to consume all of his nutrition by mouth. When he was unable to complete blocks orally, he used the NG tube. Because he did not like the sensation of bolus feeds, he became determined to eat the food and asked that the NG be removed to further motivate him. The NG was removed and did not need to be replaced. Tim was able to gradually progress to the goal of 3400 daily calories with a 10 block plan. Blocks were progressively increased until they reached 340 kcals/block, except for a smaller breakfast given that the first meal of the day had always been the most challenging.

Tim was discharged home on the Ladder Block Plan to use as a transitional tool in his home environment and was scheduled to see an outpatient OT who reinforced use of his coping strategies. The RD also taught Tim how to increase the caloric density of his favorite foods and specified which brands to purchase to maximize caloric intake. Over time, he was able to graduate from the Ladder Block Plan and was able to eat intuitively. Reflecting on his experience, he noted that having a clear plan and having accountability for practicing were the two things that helped him be successful.

Chapter 20
Fear of Aversive Consequences Case Study (Hannah)

Case Presentation

Hannah is a 13-year-old cisgender female who presents with a 10-pound weight loss from restrictive eating due to concerns about multiple food allergies (Fig. 20.1). Three months ago, Hannah experienced lip swelling and a single episode of vomiting after consuming walnut sourdough bread at a restaurant. Following that episode, her parents report several additional allergic reactions to food items with symptoms consisting of lip tingling and swelling, throat "pressure", or abdominal pain. She did not have any further episodes of vomiting. She obtained testing through an on-line, home testing company and was told that she has multiple food allergies including nuts (walnuts), fruits (coconut, cantaloupe), and certain legumes and vegetables

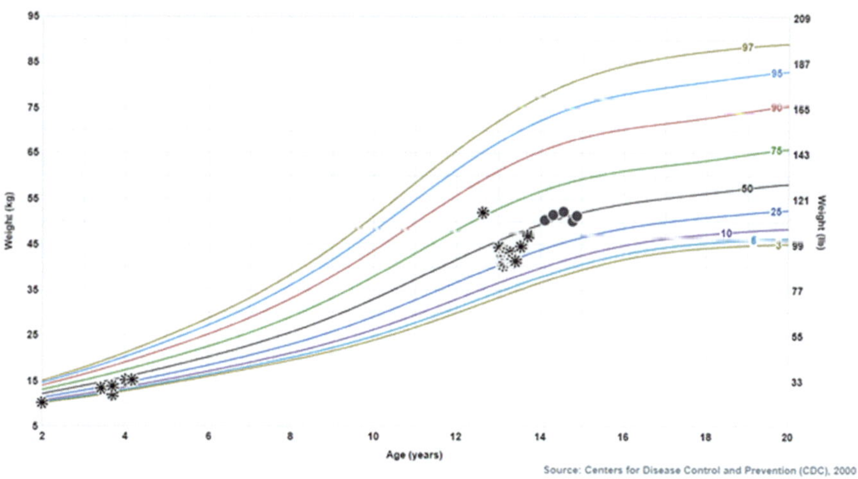

Fig. 20.1 Growth chart for Hannah

A. B. Sinha et al., *Comprehensive Clinical Care for Adolescents with Avoidant/Restrictive Food Intake Disorder (ARFID)*,
https://doi.org/10.1007/978-3-031-92232-9_20

(soy, green pea, pumpkin, onion). Her parents are very concerned about ensuring foods presented to her do not include any "unsafe" ingredients. Hannah denies body image concerns and does not want to lose weight. However, she expresses concern about having another allergic episode.

On exam, she appears thin but stable. Her vital signs are normal with a weight that is lower than her typical weight percentile.

Notable Studies include: her allergy testing IgE results indicate "high" to walnuts and "equivocal" or "low" results to all other food items noted as allergens.

Medical

Hannah's medical presentation was notable for weight loss from restricted eating. Fortunately, her vital signs and screening laboratory results were normal. As her eating concerns were very focused on avoiding subsequent allergic reactions, it was paramount to identify any true allergies. Her episode of lip swelling and vomiting was consistent with an allergic reaction. Her at-home allergen testing indicated sensitivities to a wide range of foods, though her testing performed by an allergist was notable for reactivity to only sunflower seeds (Fig. 20.2). As home allergy testing may not be accurate for diagnosing true food allergies, it is recommended to consult with an allergist to clarify an allergy diagnosis. For Hannah, her Allergist stated that only walnuts should be avoided; the other foods that she had "low" responses to were safe to continue in her diet. In addition to clarifying the allergy diagnosis, the Allergy team prescribed Hannah with an auto-injector epinephrine pen in case of any future anaphylactic reactions.

As Hannah was medically stable and working with additional team members, she was followed by the medical team at one-month intervals to ensure that she was gaining weight and remained medically stable. The medical stability determination allowed other team members to better focus their efforts. For example, if medically stable, a focus could be on incorporating challenge foods as opposed to incorporating higher volumes of safe foods. Once sustained medical progress was noted for several visits in a row, she was discharged from the medical clinic and resumed pediatric care with her primary care clinician.

Fig. 20.2 Allergy testing table for Hannah

Food	IgE	Interpretation
Garlic	**0.13**	**Equiv/Low**
Yeast	**0.26**	**Equiv/Low**
Olive, black	< 0.10	Negative
Pumpkin	**0.19**	**Equiv/Low**
Dill	< 0.10	Negative
Sweet Potato	**0.15**	**Equiv/Low**
Parsley	**0.1**	**Equiv/Low**
Melon	**0.15**	**Equiv/Low**
Mustard	< 0.10	Negative
Mango	**0.17**	**Equiv/Low**
Peach	**0.13**	**Equiv/Low**
Sole	< 0.10	Negative
Red Beet	**0.22**	**Equiv/Low**
Sunflower Seed	**2.65**	**High**
Pineapple	< 0.10	Negative
Spinach	**0.14**	**Equiv/Low**
Paprika	**0.34**	**Low**
Swordfish	< 0.10	Negative
Green Bell	< 0.10	Negative
Kidney Bean	**0.12**	**Equiv/Low**
Cauliflower	**0.17**	**Equiv/Low**
Lime	< 0.10	Negative
Chickpea	**1.29**	**Moderate**
Green Bean	**0.12**	**Equiv/Low**

Psychiatry

Hannah was seen by an eating disorder specialty psychologist to confirm the lack of body image issues. She was diagnosed with ARFID, fear of aversive consequences subtype. Parents were encouraged to take control of the renourishment process but needed a lot of education and up to date, medically sound information about allergies. During the evaluation, it was also determined that Hannah had significant generalized anxiety symptoms, including panic attacks and anticipatory anxiety around the physical symptoms heralding anaphylaxis. Her parents confirmed that multiple family members on both sides of the family struggled with anxiety symptoms, and several of them took psychotropic medications with good success. They were concerned, however, that she was too young to take psychotropic medications, and worried about the potential for having an allergy to medications.

The family responded well to education about anxiety and the impact of avoidance on inadvertently reinforcing anxiety symptoms. Their psychologist explained that it is very common to see disordered eating behaviors arise in individuals needing to avoid certain foods due to medical conditions and illustrated the hypervigilance to body sensations that can occur in these patients.

Food exposures were conducted primarily with occupational therapy, but Hannah struggled enough that the team strongly encouraged the family to consider an SSRI. She was referred to a general psychiatrist who initiated sertraline at a low dose and titrated it upward to a dose that was well tolerated and provided good symptom control (100 mg po daily in Hannah's case). The team and family agreed to continue the medications until she had been back to baseline for six to 12 months to avoid a relapse of symptoms.

Nutrition

The dietitian discovered that Hannah's main food sources were mostly limited to the following:

grains/starches: oats, rice, granola
protein: tuna, ahi tuna, salmon, chicken
fats: butter, cream, canola oil, olive oil
dairy: cheese with no soy rennet, plain yogurt
fruits and vegetables: apple juice, lettuce

With such limited variety, Hannah was estimated to be consuming about 1200–1500 calories per day, which explained her recent weight loss. The RD emphasized the importance of adequate nutrition and food expansion to help her body better tolerate foods in general. Although she was nervous, she agreed to reintroducing some foods since she reported feeling hungry and bored by her currently restrictive diet. Parents also expressed concerns around Hannah's hyperfocus on food safety. She was intently reading food labels and spending a lot of time researching foods that contain "safe" ingredients. Since the medical team had already established the safety of reintroducing foods and reassured the family that the at-home testing did not reflect true allergens, Hannah and the RD reviewed the allergy test results and highlighted the foods that were in the 0/1 category. Together, they specified which items to reintroduce: white potato, tomato, garlic, ginger, peach, parsley. The dietitian created a written meal plan to outline the following food exposures: Ginger chews, Potatoes (and then, garlic French fries), canned peaches, and cherry tomatoes.

A replacement plan was implemented in the case that Hannah was not able to fully finish the food exposure. Hannah admitted that if there was no "consequence" then she found it harder to stay motivated or committed to finishing the food exposure. An allergen free supplement was tried in session and Hannah agreed to use it for replacement.

Although calorie goals are often not explicitly discussed in many eating disorder outpatient nutrition sessions, the dietitian shared that Hannah should be eating 2600–2800 kcals/day to promote weight repletion. Hannah and her family found this information to be helpful and enlightening. The dietitian created 3 sample meal plans to exhibit how much food is needed on a 2000 calorie, 2400 calorie (Fig. 20.3), and 2800 calorie day of intake. Benecalorie, a modular with a high calorie and protein content, was mixed into Hannah's safe foods of oatmeal and apple juice to help promote weight gain at the beginning of treatment. As she continued to make progress with her food intake and demonstrated adequate weight repletion, Benecalorie was no longer needed and instead, the use of other fat sources such as oil and butter were included in her foods to increase density.

The RD made sure to thoroughly review notes from other team members and reference that information in sessions with the family. The RD also helped Hannah anticipate potential eating challenges like restaurant outings, family gatherings, and spending time at a friend's house for which they were able to brainstorm coping strategies and skills. Throughout the nutrition sessions, Hannah was able to gradually increase her intake of the identified challenge foods and the next set of items to reintroduce were worked on until Hannah felt comfortable adding back these foods on her own.

Meal Plan Image This meal plan shows how much nutrition is needed to reach 2400 kcal/day. During the hospital admission, inclusion of foods from home needed to be planned in advance so the RD knew what other foods to add to her meal/snack trays. Exposure Food items were foods that Hannah agreed to trying. Of note, replacement would be provided for those exposure foods and portions amounts were kept small and manageable to promote success with eating 100% of such foods.

2400 KCAL									
Breakfast		**Lunch**		**1400 Snack**		**Dinner**		**2000 Snack**	
FOODS FROM HOME ARE HIGHLIGHTED IN YELLOW									
****STAFF/FAMILY TO ADD TO TRAY/SNACK BAG****									
EXPOSURE FOODS IN RED - SHOULD BE REPLACED IF NOT 100% CONSUMED									
From Home: Salted Butter (1 tbsp) --> if replacement is needed, then 1 tbsp = 100 mL of Ensure Clear	100	**From Home: Salted Butter** (1 tbsp) --> if replacement is needed, then 1 tbsp = 100 mL of Ensure Clear	100	**From Home: Granola** (1/2 cup) --> if replacement is needed, then 1/2 cup = 190 mL of Ensure Clear	190	**Exposure Food:** Plain Baked Potato (1/2 potato)	40	**From Home: Popcorn** (2 cups) --> if replacement is needed, then 2 cups = 80 mL of Ensure Clear	80
Oatmeal (3/4 cup) -- ***mix with butter from home***	89	Jasmine Rice (2/3 cup) - ***mix with butter from home***	140	Greek Yogurt - Whole Milk Plain (3/4 cup)	170	Couscous (1/2 cup) -- ***mix with olive oil***	131	Whole Milk (8 oz)	160
OPTIONAL Brown Sugar (1 tbsp)		**Exposure Food:** Oil & Vinegar (1 tbsp)	70	**Exposure Food:** Canned Peaches (1/3 cup)	25	Olive Oil (1/2 tbsp)	60	Apple Slices (1 bag)	30
Banana (1 whole)	105	Plain Baked Chicken (3 oz)	140			Plain Baked Salmon (3 oz)	140		
Exposure Food: Chicken Apple Sausage (1 link)	120	Garden Green Salad - leafy greens only (3 oz)	20			Vanilla Ice Cream (1/2 cup)	130		
Whole Milk (8 oz)	160	Apple Juice (8 oz)	120			Apple Juice (8 oz)	120		
	574		590		385		621		270
								2440	

Fig. 20.3 Sample meal plan for Hannah

Occupational Therapy

The occupational therapist reviewed the pertinent medical information and confirmed that Hannah was cleared by her outpatient allergy team and adolescent medicine team to restore the foods that she had been restricting to her diet (except for tree nuts, which were deemed a true allergy).

Hannah identified her goals "to gain weight" and "eat easily again." She reported that she wanted these goals a 10/10 and was willing to work at them at a 10/10 but clarified that she was scared. She identified her barriers to full nutrition as fear of vomiting 9/10 and fear of allergic reaction to food 10/10 and fear of nausea 7/10. She reported that every time she ate, she was feeling "tingling" that reminded her of the allergic reaction. Hannah had vomited at the time of her allergic reaction episode but had not vomited since that time. At the time of the referral, the dietitian had recommended a safe supplement formula. Due to ongoing anxiety, she had only taken a couple small sips of it.

The occupational therapist privately provided education to Hannah's mother about exposures. OT encouraged parents to display confidence in Hannah's ability to tolerate a variety of foods. The OT emphasized that Hannah was going to have moments of fear and discomfort and that her parents' confidence in her ability to eat normally again would be important. She was encouraged to ask questions or share worries privately.

The occupational therapist taught Hannah and her mother the technique for avoiding vomiting (loose body posture with abdominal breathing). The OT then reviewed strategies for addressing nausea (i.e., pressure point, aromatherapy and education about the relief band). OT reinforced the importance of making these strategies readily available at the start of each eating experience. OT also taught Hannah the pressure points for early satiety since Hannah had gotten into the habit of eating small meals. After a small break, Hannah was asked to demonstrate eating preferred foods.

During the eating portion of the evaluation, Hannah was observed to have a rotary chew and normal oral motor patterns. She reported feeling full after consuming half of the oats and rice that her mother brought to the session and worried that she would vomit if she tried to eat more. She practiced abdominal breathing and pressure points in the moment to reinforce the strategies learned earlier in the session and was ultimately able to complete another quarter of the food presented. For homework, the occupational therapist encouraged Hannah to challenge herself to eat beyond fullness and to use her strategies at each meal and snack. She was also asked to practice abdominal breathing with loose body posture at least twice per day outside of her meals and snacks. Hannah and her mother agreed to this plan. The family was encouraged to bring the RD recommended nutrition supplement to the next session, which was strategically scheduled for the lunch hour.

When Hannah returned to the clinic, her family reported that she was eating 50–75% of the provided food and was practicing the strategies as recommended. She noticed that it was easier to do this at home as compared to meals that occurred at school. Hannah now reported a fear of vomiting was 5/10, fear of nausea was 4/10 and fear of allergic reaction remained 10/10. She reported that she was starting to feel more trusting that she would not vomit and more confident in her ability to handle nausea with the relief band and aromatherapy. She was wearing a relief band throughout the day, including at school. Hannah noticed that she occasionally had nausea at times other than meals. For example, it happened during a school exam or when she thought her teacher would call on her. With this information, OT helped her identify that she may have nausea at times related to anxiety.

Privately, her mother reported that Hannah seemed less anxious and was less resistant to eating but still wasn't eating enough. She had been using the strategies consistently and her mom did not think Hannah was nearly as nervous about vomiting anymore. Collaboratively, they brainstormed incentives to reward Hannah for her hard work on increasing eating and consuming the supplementation and shared a behavior modification chart with Hannah. Hannah was excited about the potential to earn money she could spend on toys and treats for her puppy.

After a quick break, lunch was started. Because the session was limited to an hour, the OT was careful to reassure Hannah that she would not be rushed to complete the entire meal in the time remaining. OT had the patient taste test the supplement first. Hannah ranked the appearance as a 3/5, the texture as a 3/5, the taste as a 4/5 and the "like it" as a 3/5 and reported that she felt she could drink it. OT encouraged her to take sips of it throughout the meal so that she would complete the full 1 ounce during the meal. Hannah ate at a moderate pace and took small sips. At 15 min into the meal, she reported fullness and had completed 60% of her food. OT encouraged her to get to at least 75% + to get more points and to complete her supplement. Hannah was able to do both and completed 90% of her nutrition. OT had her fill out her points on the behavioral modification sheet and requested that she do so at each meal and snack (outside of school) and that she bring it back at the next session. Hannah's mom was encouraged to increase the amount of supplement presented at each meal and snack by one ounce up to a goal of four ounces. The supplement could be increased once Hannah was able to consistently complete her supplement as requested for 1–2 days.

At the next session, OT reviewed progress with the family and worked to troubleshoot any problems. For example, Hannah was encouraged to challenge herself to wake up 15 min earlier in the morning and set out clothes the night before so that she didn't run out of time to complete her breakfast before school. They reviewed and reinforced the behavioral modification plan and celebrated Hannah's successes together (Hannah was excited about the dog toy she was planning to purchase on the way home from the session). They also continued to review and practice coping strategies, and Hannah shared the real-life experiences she had using them. Privately, Hannah's mother shared that Hannah was less apprehensive and was eating more but expanding her food repertoire seemed to be the last remaining issue. In preparation for this next phase of treatment, OT reviewed the food exploration document that would be used at the next session. Because the goal of the upcoming food exploration was not to focus on the texture or taste of the food, but to help Hannah observe that she tended to have anxiety related symptoms before, during and after eating, the occupational therapist had modified the typically used food exploration log to help her observe her sensations before and after eating. A plan was made to trial a potato at the next session.

At the next session, the OT was intentional about reviewing the goals of the session and reassuring Hannah that her doctor felt that it was safe to trial eating a potato. She was given a short break before the exposure. Mom also happily consumed a potato during the session to reinforce the sentiment that everyone was confident and excited about the challenge. Hannah was asked to formally observe her sensation levels (Fig. 20.4), including prior to starting to eat. She reported that

Food name	Sensation level before	Sensation level after	Any observations?	Trial #
Potato	3 lips, nose, belly	3 belly, lips	Same	1

Fig. 20.4 Hannah's food exploration log result examining sensations pre and post eating perceived allergen

she felt sensation (tingling) in her lips, nose, and belly at 3/10. After consuming a slice of potato in 3+ bites, Hannah noted that she still felt a 3/10 tingling now only in her belly and lips, not in her nose. Hannah was able to notice that she had the same sensations before and after eating the food.

After a short break, the occupational therapist asked the patient if she had any thoughts about what it meant if she had the same sensations before and after eating the potato. Hannah reported that she was not sure what that meant but thought it might mean that it was not an allergic reaction. The OT reviewed that the patient had gotten into an unhelpful pattern after her allergic reaction. She reviewed that it was going to require practice eating previously consumed foods to get confident with eating them again and that, over time, she would no longer have sensation around eating them.

OT asked the patient again on a scale of 1–10 how much she "wanted to eat normally again." Hannah reported that it was still a 10/10. The OT asked the patient how much she was willing to work at it. Hannah reported that it was still a 10/10 but that she felt nervous sometimes. The occupational therapist encouraged Hannah to practice her abdominal breathing not only for avoiding nausea, but also at times if she felt nervous. Hannah agreed to do this. The occupational therapist modified Hannah's behavior modification plan to reflect her current eating goals and added points for taking 3+ bites of "newer foods" (i.e., foods she hadn't eaten for awhile) at home. The OT requested that Hannah have potatoes at least once per day after school and at least one weekend day each week. The OT requested that her mom and Hannah pick out two previously consumed foods to bring to the next session to continue food exploration. OT continued the exposure (soybeans and garlic string beans) at the next session. Hannah continued to gradually progress in her treatment and "practices" within and outside of the OT treatment sessions.

Treatment culminated in food exploration activities during which Hannah was able to identify sensations and worries before and after exposures that allowed her to see that she was indeed not experiencing an allergic reaction. This was an essential experience that allowed her to reintroduce previously enjoyed foods. After a couple positive and successful experiences of exposures and observations, Hannah and her mom felt more confident and continued to do explorations at home until Hannah returned to her prior eating baseline. At discharge, Hannah's fear of an allergic reaction diminished to 2/10 and she felt confident that she knew how to avoid vomiting. She also felt confident in her techniques for addressing anxiety. She still occasionally had sensations, but acknowledged that they were related to her worry thoughts and she did not let them influence her eating. At that point, after 12 treatment sessions over a 6 month period, Hannah was discharged from outpatient occupational therapy.

Chapter 21
Conclusion

Even though the diagnosis of ARFID was new to the DSM-5 in 2013, the features that make up the diagnosis have been present long before that. Increased awareness of the existence of ARFID has resulted in better identification and more individuals and their families seeking treatment. With this formal diagnosis comes opportunities for ongoing treatment design and research to determine gold standard practices It is our belief that ARFID treatment is most successful when it is customized to the individual. While ARFID and other restrictive eating disorders can result in malnutrition, the process, type, and execution of the nutrition plan is incredibly individualized and varied. Moreover, there is a difference in presentations amongst ARFID subtypes and patients within each subtype or subtypes can have specific needs.

Correctly diagnosing ARFID and determining the appropriate ARFID subtype(s) and features can guide practitioners in the best possible treatment approach. Addressing perceived barriers to nutrition prior to doing feeding sessions with patients is critical for helping the patient shift out of their behavioral patterns around food. Regardless of what a patient identifies as their barriers, eating with patients is an important component of effective treatment. When treatment members eat with patients, often additional barriers are discovered (e.g., oral motor barriers, postural barriers, bite size, etc.) that the patient may not have identified. Repeatedly eating with patients can help them address their barriers and shift their patterns for more effective eating. Family members are the most important team members in supporting the patient in feeding. Providing family training to optimize patient support and intake is an important component for helping patients change their eating patterns.

A multidisciplinary approach in treating ARFID is ideal, and experienced providers can make all the difference in treatment outcomes. In addition to including medical and mental health providers with eating disorder experience, working with a dietitian who understands the ARFID subtypes is important. For example, if there is an ARFID- sensory subtype patient who is of low weight and only eats less than a dozen foods, the dietitian can work with them on how to optimize their current

A. B. Sinha et al., *Comprehensive Clinical Care for Adolescents with Avoidant/Restrictive Food Intake Disorder (ARFID)*,
https://doi.org/10.1007/978-3-031-92232-9_21

food preferences by focusing on density and/or frequency, whereas if the individual is ARFID- sensory subtype of normal weight, the dietitian may first focus on food exploration and expansion. While feeding occupational therapists or speech therapists are known to treat ARFID patients in the outpatient world, they are not consistently included in inpatient and residential treatment programs. Their contribution and unique approach is an asset when serving ARFID patients as many patients have unaddressed oral motor or postural patterns impacting their feeding and their clinical practice areas include feeding and a study of physiology. When occupational therapists (or STs) make and modify behavior modification plans based on the patients' presentation during feeding, progress can be amplified and become integrated in their lives. Finally, patients with co-occurring conditions such as anxiety or other psychiatric diagnoses may benefit from working with a psychiatric prescriber who has familiarity with treating this patient population.

Prioritizing the patient's needs is imperative. This includes understanding the severity of their medical condition as well as what will be required for the patient to return to a place of health. After learning strategies, the first goal for most ARFID patients is increasing their nutrition intake through any means. If they are at a low weight or have a nutrient deficiency, the next priorities are to be able to get nutrition through a supplement, to resume previously consumed foods, expand the food repertoire, and to be able to take in adequate nutrition in a range of settings.

We hope that after reading this book you recognize the value of a multidisciplinary team in addressing ARFID, the significance of understanding and recognizing the ARFID subtypes to guide treatment and the importance of working closely with the family in order to capitalize on their expertise in their child and family. There is much yet to be learned and studied about these patients, but we feel confident that treatment approaches will continue to be refined and improved over time.

Chapter 22
Clinical Tools and Protocols

A. B. Sinha et al., *Comprehensive Clinical Care for Adolescents with Avoidant/Restrictive Food Intake Disorder (ARFID)*,
https://doi.org/10.1007/978-3-031-92232-9_22

Nutrition Appendix (Allyson SY)

Appendix 1: The 5 Food Guide

THE 5 FOOD GUIDE©

NAME: ____________ DATE: ____________

Instructions
For each food item, please color code each item according to your preference:

- **Red** - foods you dislike and cannot eat
- **Yellow** - foods you're indifferent/neutral towards (you don't love it but don't dislike it) and can sometimes eat
- **Green** - foods you love and can eat
- **Blue** - foods you used to like or eat but not currently eating
- **Purple**- foods you've never eaten and want to try

Write down any specifics about any of the food items (such as brand names, types, how it's made or prepared, food pairings, etc) in the "Comments" column. While this list is long, it does not capture all of the foods in every category so please write down any other foods that are missing that you feel is important to write about.

Grains/Starches	Comments
Oatmeal, Overnight Oats Cream of Wheat, Cream of Rice	
Granola, Muesli	
Bread, English Muffin, Bagel	
Cereal	
Biscuit, Croissant, Scone	
Baked Goods, Muffins, Donuts	
Pancakes. French Toast, Waffles	
Crepes: Sweet, Savory	

THE 5 FOOD GUIDE©

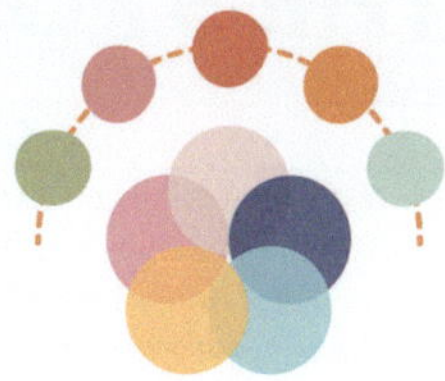

Color Key:

- **Red** – foods you dislike and cannot eat
- **Yellow** – foods you're indifferent/neutral towards (you don't love it but don't dislike it) and can sometimes eat
- **Green** – foods you love and can eat
- **Blue** – foods you used to like or eat but not currently eating
- **Purple**– foods you've never eaten and want to try

Grains/Starches	Comments
Potatoes: Baked, Mashed, Diced, Roasted	
Hash Browns, Tater Tots, French Fries	
Rice	
Rice Porridge, Fried Rice	
Noodles	
Pasta	
Couscous, Quinoa, Barley	
Polenta, Cornmeal	
Tortilla	
Roti. Naan	

THE 5 FOOD GUIDE©

Color Key:
• **Red** – foods you dislike and cannot eat • **Yellow** – foods you're indifferent/neutral towards (you don't love it but don't dislike it) and can sometimes eat • **Green** – foods you love and can eat • **Blue** – foods you used to like or eat but not currently eating • **Purple**– foods you've never eaten and want to try

Protein	Comments
Beef: Steak, Ground Beef, Deli Meat, Bacon Sausages, Links, Hot Dog	
Chicken: Roasted, Fried, Ground Chicken Chicken Nuggets/Tenders, Deli Meat Sausages, Links, Hot Dog	
Pork: Pork Loin, Ground Pork, Deli Meat, Bacon Sausages, Links, Hot Dog, Spam	
Turkey: Roasted, Ground Turkey, Deli Meat, Bacon Sausages, Links, Hot Dog	
Fish: Salmon, Mahi Mahi, Tuna , Cod, Halibut Catfish, Tilapia, Fish Sticks	
Shellfish: Shrimp, Prawns, Crab, Lobster, Clams Mussels, Oysters, Scallop, Calamari	
Lamb, Duck, Goat	
Eggs: Scrambled, Omelette, Hard Boiled Over Easy, Poached, Sunny Side Up	
Nuts, Nut Butters* **Also can be considered a source of* ***Fats***	

THE 5 FOOD GUIDE©

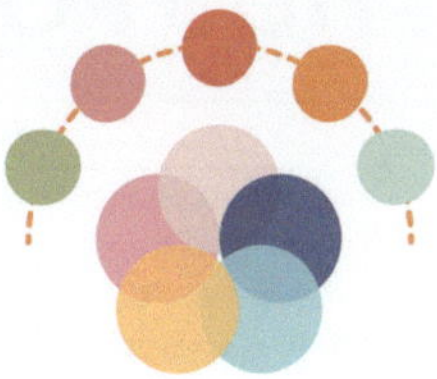

Color Key:
• **Red** – foods you dislike and cannot eat • **Yellow** – foods you're indifferent/neutral towards (you don't love it but don't dislike it) and can sometimes eat • **Green** – foods you love and can eat • **Blue** – foods you used to like or eat but not currently eating • **Purple**– foods you've never eaten and want to try

Protein	Comments
Beans: Pinto, Black, Kidney, White, Refried	
Peas, Edamame, Lentils	
Chickpeas, Hummus	

Dairy/Dairy Alternatives*	Comments
*Also can be considered a source of ***Protein***	
Milk: Whole, 2%, 1%, Fat Free Chocolate, Strawberry	
Yogurt, Yogurt Drinks, Kefir	
Cheese: Sliced, Shredded	
Cottage Cheese	
Ice Cream, Ice Cream Bars, Frozen Yogurt	
Milkshakes	

THE 5 FOOD GUIDE©

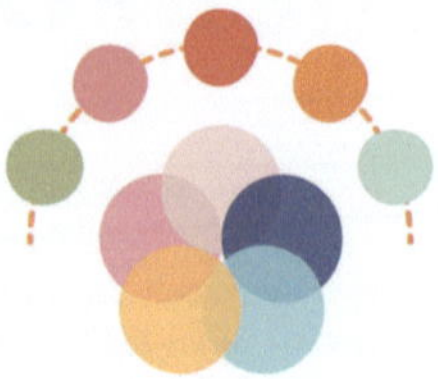

Color Key:
• **Red** – foods you dislike and cannot eat • **Yellow** – foods you're indifferent/neutral towards (you don't love it but don't dislike it) and can sometimes eat • **Green** – foods you love and can eat • **Blue** – foods you used to like or eat but not currently eating • **Purple**– foods you've never eaten and want to try

Fruits	Comments
Apples: Applesauce, Dried Fruit, Juice	
Bananas, Plantains	
Grapes, Raisins, Juice	
Mangoes, Dried Fruit, Juice	
Pineapple, Dried Fruit, Juice	
Melons: Cantaloupe, Honeydew, Watermelon	
Berries: Strawberry, Blueberry, Raspberry Blackberry, Cranberry Dried Fruit, Juice	
Oranges, Tangerines, Juice	
Pear, Peach, Nectarine, Apricot Dried Fruit	
Persimmons	
Lemon, Lime, Juice	
Mixed Fruit Cup, Canned Fruit	
Fruit Snacks, Fruit Belts, Fruit Bars	
Smoothies, Smoothie Bowls	

THE 5 FOOD GUIDE©

Color Key:

- **Red** – foods you dislike and cannot eat
- **Yellow** – foods you're indifferent/neutral towards (you don't love it but don't dislike it) and can sometimes eat
- **Green** – foods you love and can eat
- **Blue** – foods you used to like or eat but not currently eating
- **Purple**– foods you've never eaten and want to try

Vegetables	Comments
Lettuce, Salad Greens	
Spinach, Kale, Collard Greens	
Broccoli, Broccolini, Cauliflower	
Potato, Sweet Potato, Yam* **Also can be considered a source of* ***Grains/Starches***	
Carrots, Baby Carrots	
Tomatoes	
Corn, Peas	
Mushrooms	
Green Beans	
Bell Peppers, Mini Peppers	
Acorn Squash, Butternut Squash	
Zucchini	
Eggplant	
Celery	
Beets	
Artichoke, Brussel Sprouts	
Onions, Garlic	

THE 5 FOOD GUIDE©

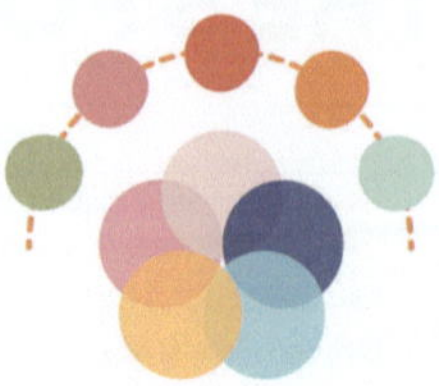

Color Key:
• **Red** – foods you dislike and cannot eat • **Yellow** – foods you're indifferent/neutral towards (you don't love it but don't dislike it) and can sometimes eat • **Green** – foods you love and can eat • **Blue** – foods you used to like or eat but not currently eating • **Purple**– foods you've never eaten and want to try

Fats	Comments
Avocado, Guacamole	
Olives	
Butter, Margarine, Ghee	
Oils	
Salad Dressing	
Cream Cheese	
Sour Cream	
Mayonaisse	
Gravy	
Sesame Seeds, Tahini	
Dips	
Coconut Milk	

THE 5 FOOD GUIDE©

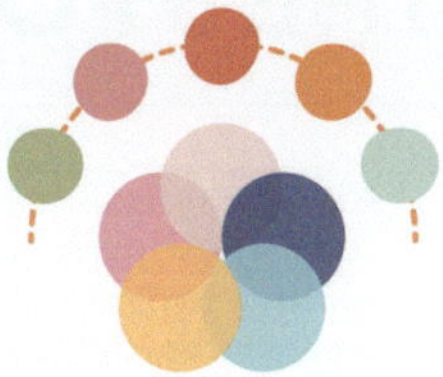

Color Key:
• **Red** – foods you dislike and cannot eat • **Yellow** – foods you're indifferent/neutral towards (you don't love it but don't dislike it) and can sometimes eat • **Green** – foods you love and can eat • **Blue** – foods you used to like or eat but not currently eating • **Purple**– foods you've never eaten and want to try

Instructions:
Add more foods to the "Main Entrees" list if an important food is not already listed below. Color code each item according to your liking. Write down any important notes about the food (such as brand names, types, how it's made or prepared, etc) under the "Comments" section.

Main Entrees	Comments
Sandwiches	
Burgers	
Wraps	
Pizza	
Burritos, Tacos	
Soup	
Pasta	
Sushi	

THE 5 FOOD GUIDE©

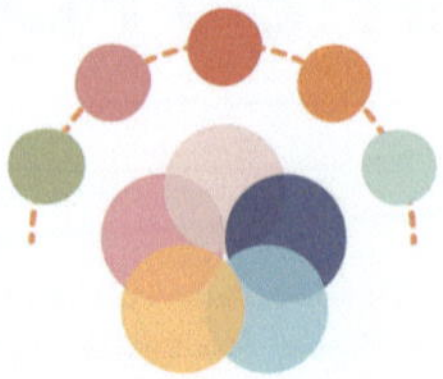

Color Key:

- **Red** – foods you dislike and cannot eat
- **Yellow** – foods you're indifferent/neutral towards (you don't love it but don't dislike it) and can sometimes eat
- **Green** – foods you love and can eat
- **Blue** – foods you used to like or eat but not currently eating
- **Purple**– foods you've never eaten and want to try

Instructions:

Add more foods to the "Snacks, Sweets, Dessert" list if an important food is not already listed below.
Color code each item according to your liking.
Write down any important notes about the food (such as brand names, types, how it's made or prepared, etc) under the "Comments" section.

Snacks, Sweets, Dessert	Comments
Chips	
Crackers	
Pretzels	
Granola Bars, Protein Bars	
Candy	
Chocolate	
Cake, Cheesecake	
Pie	
Cookies	

THE 5 FOOD GUIDE©

Color Key:

- **Red** – foods you dislike and cannot eat
- **Yellow** – foods you're indifferent/neutral towards (you don't love it but don't dislike it) and can sometimes eat
- **Green** – foods you love and can eat
- **Blue** – foods you used to like or eat but not currently eating
- **Purple**– foods you've never eaten and want to try

Instructions:

Add more foods to the "Beverages" and "Other Foods" list if an important food is not already listed below.
Color code each item according to your liking.
Write down any important notes about the food (such as brand names, types, how it's made or prepared, etc) under the "Comments" section.

Beverages	Comments
Juice	
Coffee, Hot Chocolate, Tea	
Water, Sparkling Water	
Soda	
Smoothies	

Other Foods	Comments

Appendix 2: The 5 Food Basic Guide

THE 5 FOOD GUIDE©

NAME: ____________ **DATE:** ____________

Instructions
Color code each food item according to your liking: • **Red** – foods you dislike and cannot eat • **Yellow** – foods you're indifferent/neutral towards (you don't love it but don't dislike it) and can sometimes eat • **Green** – foods you love and can eat • **Blue** – foods you used to like or eat but not currently eating • **Purple**– foods you've never eaten and want to try Write down any important notes about the food (such as brand names, types, how it's made or prepared, etc) under the "Comments" section.

Grains/Starches	Comments
Oatmeal	
Granola	
Cereal	
Bread	
Pancakes, Waffles, French Toast	
Rice	
Potatoes	
Pasta	
Noodles	
Tortilla	
Gluten-Free	

THE 5 FOOD GUIDE©

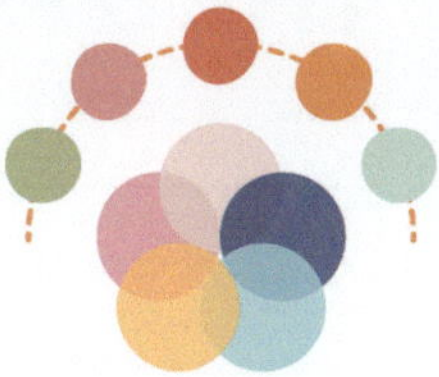

Color Key:
• **Red** – foods you dislike and cannot eat • **Yellow** – foods you're indifferent/neutral towards (you don't love it but don't dislike it) and can sometimes eat • **Green** – foods you love and can eat • **Blue** – foods you used to like or eat but not currently eating • **Purple**– foods you've never eaten and want to try

Protein	Comments
Chicken	
Beef	
Pork	
Turkey	
Fish, Seafood	
Beans, Lentils, Peas	
Eggs	
Tofu, Soybeans	
Nuts, Nut Butters	

Dairy/Dairy Alternatives	Comments
Milk	
Yogurt, Yogurt Drinks, Kefir	
Cheese, Cottage Cheese	
Ice Cream, Frozen Yogurt	
Milkshakes	

THE 5 FOOD GUIDE©

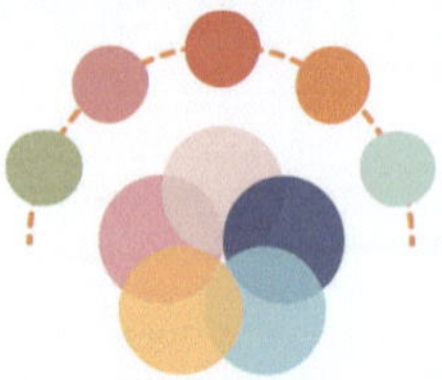

Color Key:
• **Red** – foods you dislike and cannot eat • **Yellow** – foods you're indifferent/neutral towards (you don't love it but don't dislike it) and can sometimes eat • **Green** – foods you love and can eat • **Blue** – foods you used to like or eat but not currently eating • **Purple**– foods you've never eaten and want to try

Fruit	Comments
Apples	
Bananas	
Oranges	
Grapes	
Strawberry, Blueberry, Raspberry, Blackberry, Cranberry	
Mango, Pineapple	
Cantaloupe, Honeydew, Watermelon	
Lemon, Lime	
Pear, Peach, Apricot, Nectarine	
Mixed Fruit Cup, Canned Fruit	
Fruit Snacks, Fruit Belts, Fruit Bars	
Dried Fruit	

THE 5 FOOD GUIDE©

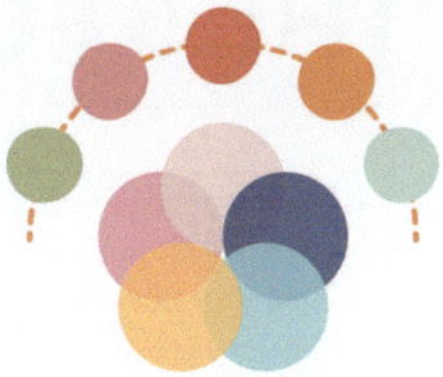

Color Key:
• **Red** – foods you dislike and cannot eat • **Yellow** – foods you're indifferent/neutral towards (you don't love it but don't dislike it) and can sometimes eat • **Green** – foods you love and can eat • **Blue** – foods you used to like or eat but not currently eating • **Purple**– foods you've never eaten and want to try

Vegetables	Comments
Broccoli, Cauliflower	
Potato, Sweet Potato	
Carrots, Baby Carrots	
Tomatoes	
Corn	
Peas	
Green Beans	
Bell Peppers, Mini Peppers	
Lettuce, Salad Greens	
Spinach, Kale	
Squash	
Zucchini	
Celery	
Mushrooms	

THE 5 FOOD GUIDE©

Color Key:
• **Red** – foods you dislike and cannot eat • **Yellow** – foods you're indifferent/neutral towards (you don't love it but don't dislike it) and can sometimes eat • **Green** – foods you love and can eat • **Blue** – foods you used to like or eat but not currently eating • **Purple**– foods you've never eaten and want to try

Fats	Comments
Avocado, Guacamole	
Olives	
Butter, Margarine, Ghee	
Oils	
Salad Dressings	
Cream Cheese	
Sour Cream	
Mayonnaise	
Gravy	
Sesame Seeds, Tahini	

THE 5 FOOD GUIDE©

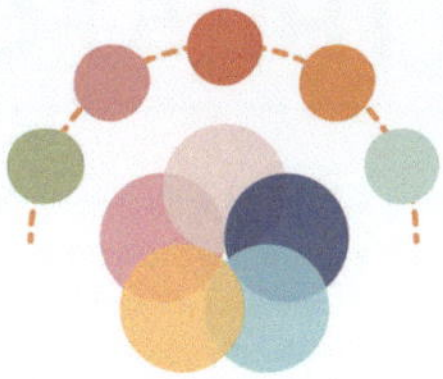

Color Key:
• **Red** – foods you dislike and cannot eat • **Yellow** – foods you're indifferent/neutral towards (you don't love it but don't dislike it) and can sometimes eat • **Green** – foods you love and can eat • **Blue** – foods you used to like or eat but not currently eating • **Purple**– foods you've never eaten and want to try

Instructions:
Add more foods to the "Main Entrees" list if an important food is not already listed below. Color code each item according to your liking. Write down any important notes about the food (such as brand names, types, how it's made or prepared, etc) under the "Comments" section.

Main Entrees	Comments
Sandwich	
Pizza	
Burger	
Sushi	
Burritos, Tacos	
Soup	
Pasta	
Chicken Tenders	

THE 5 FOOD GUIDE©

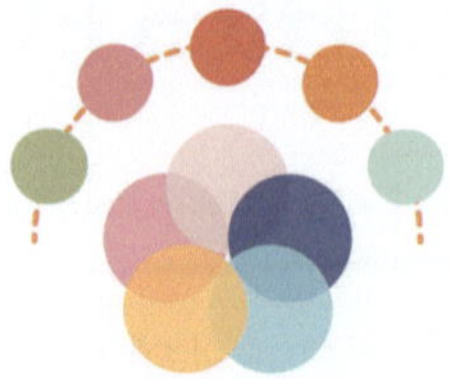

Color Key:

- **Red** – foods you dislike and cannot eat
- **Yellow** – foods you're indifferent/neutral towards (you don't love it but don't dislike it) and can sometimes eat
- **Green** – foods you love and can eat
- **Blue** – foods you used to like or eat but not currently eating
- **Purple**– foods you've never eaten and want to try

Instructions:

Add more foods to the "Snacks, Sweets, Dessert" list if an important food is not already listed below.
Color code each item according to your liking.
Write down any important notes about the food (such as brand names, types, how it's made or prepared, etc) under the "Comments" section.

Snacks, Sweets, Dessert	Comments
Chips	
Crackers	
Pretzels	
Granola Bars, Protein Bars	
Candy	
Chocolate	
Cake	
Pie	
Cookies	

THE 5 FOOD GUIDE©

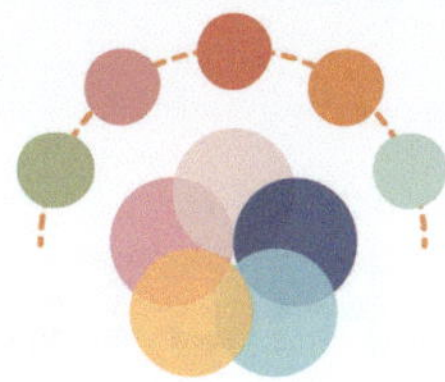

Color Key:
• **Red** – foods you dislike and cannot eat • **Yellow** – foods you're indifferent/neutral towards (you don't love it but don't dislike it) and can sometimes eat • **Green** – foods you love and can eat • **Blue** – foods you used to like or eat but not currently eating • **Purple**– foods you've never eaten and want to try

Instructions:
Add more foods to the "Beverages" and "Other Foods" lists if an important food is not already listed below. Color code each item according to your liking. Write down any important notes about the food (such as brand names, types, how it's made or prepared, etc) under the "Comments" section.

Beverages	Comments
Juice	
Coffee, Hot Chocolate, Tea	
Water, Sparkling Water	
Soda	
Smoothies	

Other Foods	Comments

Appendix 3: Picture the Plate

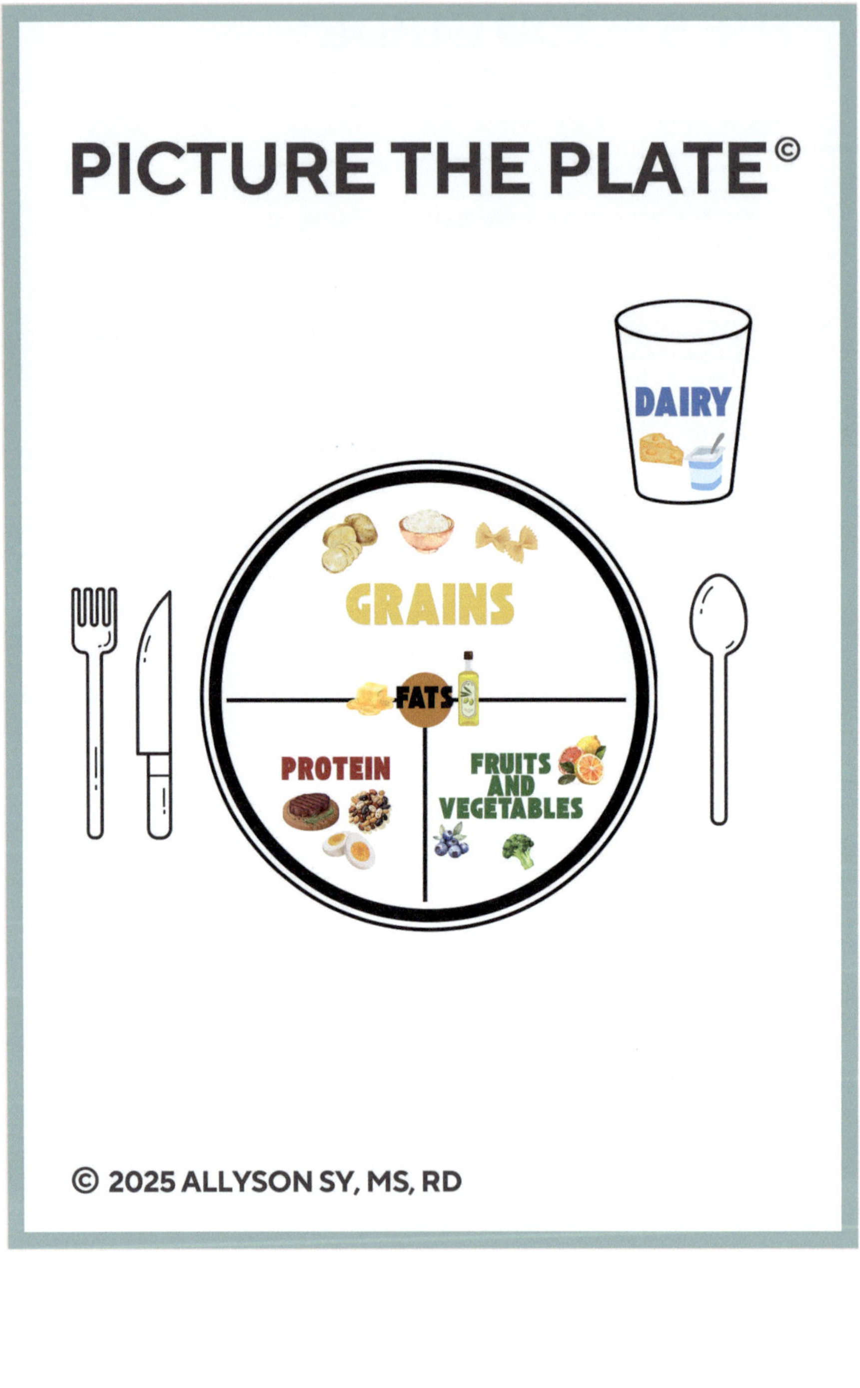

Appendix 4: Picture the One Third Plate

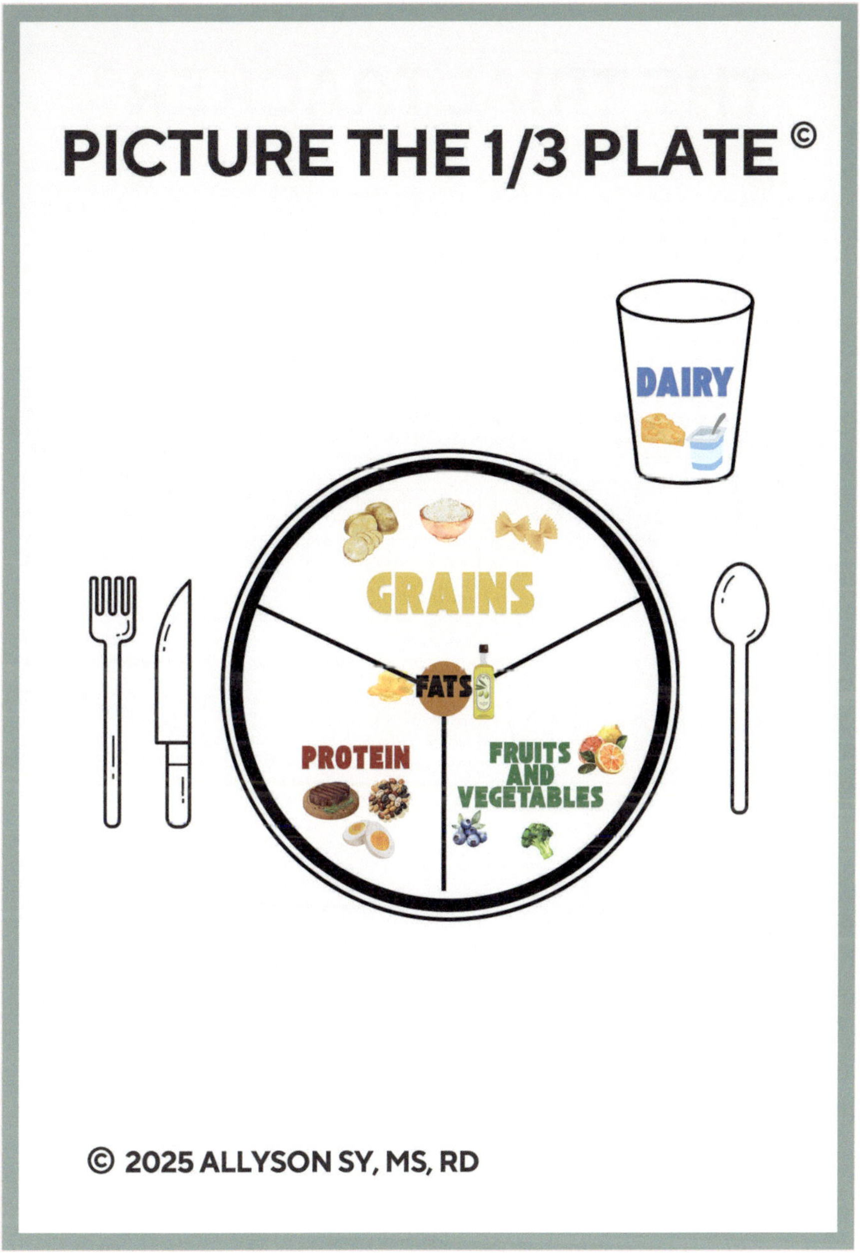

Appendix 5: The Trial Tracker

THE TRIAL TRACKER©

NAME: ____________ **DATE:** ____________

Instructions
For each food item that you try, rank how challenging that food item can be by using a scale of 1 to 10 (with "1" being "not challenging at all" and "10" being "the most challenging"). Note: the ranking of a trial food item can change when it's tried a different time. Indicate how much of the food was eaten. In the "Notes" section, describe your overall experience when trying this food. Use your five senses to help guide your exploration about the food. Comment on appearance, flavor, texture, smell, how it sounds, and how you liked it overall.

Nº	TRIAL FOOD	RANKING	AMOUNT EATEN	NOTES
1				
2				
3				
4				
5				

Appendix 6: BMod Plan Example 1

DAY: ________________ **DATE:** ________________

MEAL: ________________________

Food Trial (up to 2 per meal) Food #1: ____________________ *Circle which applies:* New Reintroduced Challenge Took 3 bites (1) Took 5 bites (2) Finished 50% (4) Finished 100% (5)	Food #2: ____________________ *Circle which applies:* New Reintroduced Challenge Took 3 bites (1) Took 5 bites (2) Finished 50% (4) Finished 100% (5)
Ate at least 75% of meal (+1 BONUS POINT)	Coping Skills Used: (+1 BONUS POINT for each one used) -Counter thought for fear (on index cards) -Deep breathing -Use of fidget toy -Visualization -Distraction techniques (engaging in game/convo, describing object) -Nonjudgment towards body sensations and emotions. -Safe space

TOTAL POINTS:

SNACK: ________________________

Food Trial (up to 2 per meal) Food #1: ____________________ *Circle which applies:* New Reintroduced Challenge Took 3 bites (1) Took 5 bites (2) Finished 25% (3) Finished 50% (4)	Food #2: ____________________ *Circle which applies:* New Reintroduced Challenge Took 3 bites (1) Took 5 bites (2) Finished 25% (3) Finished 50% (4)
Ate at least 75% of snack (+1 BONUS POINT)	Coping Skills Used: (+1 BONUS POINT for each one used) -Counter thought for fear (on index cards) -Deep breathing -Use of fidget toy -Visualization -Distraction techniques (engaging in game/convo, describing object) -Nonjudgment towards body sensations and emotions. -Safe space

TOTAL POINTS:

Appendix 7: BMod Plan Example 2

Daily routine to support wellness		
Self care goals	**Morning routine:** Wake up at 8:00 AM, get out of bed at 8:30 AM, and eat breakfast at 8:45 AM (10 pts) **Medications:** Take vitamins and meds in the morning (5 pts)	**BONUS:** Behavioral Activation/Social Activity (10 pts) **Brushing teeth:** AM (5 pts) PM (5 pts)
Breakfast	Meal has 5 food groups (5 pts)	Ate 50% (5 pts) Ate 75% (10 pts) Ate 100% (20 pts)
Mid AM snack	2 item snack at 10:30 AM (20 pts)	
Lunch	Meal has 5 food groups (5 pts)	Ate 50% or below (3 pts) Ate 75% (8 pts) Ate 100% (15 pts)
Afternoon snack	Ate 1 item* snack (2 pt) Ate 2 items of snack (4 pt) Ate 3 items of the snack** (6 pt)	**3 item snack can be an ice cream sandwich + juice *NOTE: 1 item means 1 full serving of that snack food.
Dinner	Meal has 5 food groups (5 pts)	Ate 50% or below (3 pts) Ate 75% (8 pts) Ate 100% (15 pts)
Evening snack	Ate 1 item* snack (2 pt) Ate 2 items of snack (4 pt) Ate 3 items of the snack** (6 pt)	**3 item snack can be an ice cream sandwich + juice *NOTE: 1 item means 1 full serving of that snack food.
	DAILY TOTAL POINTS: ________ **COMMENTS/OBSERVATIONS:**	

Occupational Therapy Appendix

Appendix A: Introduction to Physiological Recovery Model

For patients who are dangerously losing weight or are hospitalized, it can be helpful to review the concept of physiological recovery from malnutrition. You might explain it to patients with something like this (Fig. 22.1):

> Regardless of how it started, when the body spends too much time with too little nutrition and too much activity, even breathing can be too much if nutrition is too low. The body starts to conserve energy by changing how it functions. This can lead to reduced blood flow to the hands, feet, and head. Mood might be affected, and the heart can slow down at night to save energy. When standing up too quickly, some patients feel dizzy or faint (orthostasis), and many notice lower energy or endurance.
>
> The quickest way to recover from malnutrition is through what we call 'physiological recovery mode,' where the focus is on getting enough nutrition at regular intervals while limiting activity. In the hospital, this often starts with bedrest, and as patients improve, they gradually regain activity until they are stable enough to go home. Once home, patients typically check in with their doctors weekly to monitor progress and stability. Over time, as health improves, these visits become less frequent until they are fully recovered and only need annual check-ups.

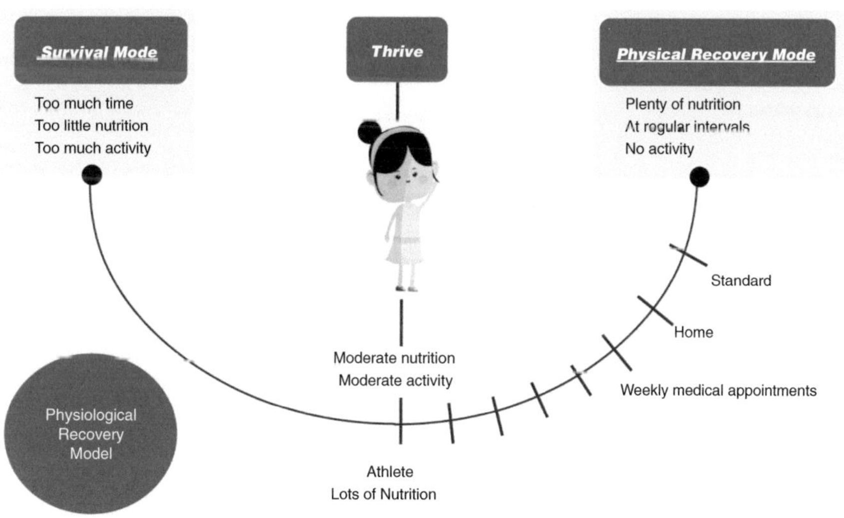

Fig. 22.1 Physiological recovery model

Appendix B: Inpatient Sample Occupational Therapy Evaluation Template

Occupational Therapy Evaluation

(fill in areas with * but all areas may require editing as this is an inpatient hospitalization sample)**

NAME: **DOB:** **MRN:** **LOC:**

Admitting Service: **Admission Date:**

Attending: **PCP:**

Date of Service: **Session Time:** *** minutes direct

OT Orders

(From admission, onward)

Complexity of this OT evaluation: Medium (sample, modify as needed)

- *Review of Medical History, & Therapy History:* ***1-2 personal factors and/or comorbidities
- *Examination of Body Systems* (elements include body structures and functions, activity limitations, and/or participation restrictions): ***1-2 elements
- Cardiovascular/pulmonary (Reference: the assessment of heart rate, respiratory rate, blood pressure, edema)
- *Clinical Presentation:* ***Evolving
- Level of Complexity for Clinical Decision Making: *** Medium

ASSESSMENT: ***

Identification / Chief Complaint

***

Patient History

***

Social History

Home Environment: Lives with ***

School: ***

Skilled Services Received: ***

Home Equipment: ***

Activity Order:

Activity Orders (From admission, onward) ***

Precautions:

***

Initial Presentation

Physical Appearance: ***

Physiological Stability: ***

Mental Status: ***

Pain Assessment:

***/10

Development:

***

Neuromotor Exam

***

Muscle Tone:

***

Coordination:

***

Functional Mobility:

***

Balance:

***

Posture:

***

Endurance: ***

Activities of Daily Living:

Currently requires supervision for adequate nutrition

***

Patient/Caregiver Education: Please see education section in chart for details

Problem List

At risk for deconditioning

Decreased ability to self-regulate

Decreased activity tolerance

Decreased endurance

Decreased caregiver knowledge

Decreased patient knowledge

Decreased knowledge of relaxation techniques

***

Goals:

Patient Goals

***

Time Frame: ***

Plan:

5/ week***

Outpatient OT***

Interventions Planned

Activities of daily living training

Community re-integration management training***

Coping skills/Relaxation training

Pain management***

Patient/Caregiver education

Positioning

***

Treatment plan established with patient/caregiver

***

Recommended Therapy Equipment for Discharge

***

Recommended Therapy Services after Discharge

- Occupational Therapy ***

Recommended Special Services and Community Resources After Discharge

***

Note created by: Name with credentials, date

Appendix C: Treating Rumination

To help patients gradually reduce the duration and frequency of rumination, an initial goal may be to extend the time without rumination beyond their baseline. For example if they typically ruminate upon completing their last bite, this could involve delaying rumination by at least 2 min after eating, with the goal of gradually increasing this time. Conscious attention on abdominal breathing with loose body posture (including no jaw tension and sightly soft or open lips) is impactful. Learning to consciously avoid rumination often requires multiple sessions and typically first involves delay. As individuals learn to delay rumination and ultimately shift the pattern, they retrain their body in preventing the food from coming up. A simple reminder that they "spent years" without the food coming up is often helpful.

A tool that can be useful in teaching rumination delay and prevention is an extra snack session of a patient-chosen quantity of nuts (without fluids). Nuts are particularly useful because their chunky and sharp texture makes them less comfortable to ruminate, and the absence of fluids further assists in managing the behavior. This extra session can be useful for any patient experiencing rumination, both ARFID and AN-R patients. Refer to Appendix L to see treatment orders appropriate for rumination patients

Appendix D: Addressing Constipation & Bowel Health Hand-Out

Addressing Constipation

Occupational therapists are well-suited to address the physiological aspects of constipation and how daily routines impact bowel health. There is a known correlation between constipation and malnutrition, making it likely that patients admitted to the hospital for malnutrition will also experience constipation. Additionally, some individuals, particularly those with ARFID-low interest or ARFID-sensory subtypes, may have had a lifelong tendency toward constipation.

Before addressing constipation, the occupational therapist can discuss with the patient how, as they grow older, they take on more responsibility for understanding, communicating about, and managing what is happening in their body. While parents often manage these details during early childhood, adolescence is a time of increasing awareness and responsibility. Though some patients may be hesitant to talk about their bowel health, it is an important responsibility of their medical team to assist the patient in comfortably having these conversations that support their long-term health.

Components of Bowel Health

When providing education about constipation, it is helpful to explain to the patient that there are three main components of bowel health (Fig. 22.2):

1. Stool is soft enough to push.
2. Toilet sitting at the right time.
3. Right coordination.

1. **Stool Soft Enough to Push:**

   Introduce patients to the Bristol Stool Chart as a tool to help them become more aware of their bowel movements and as a method of communication with their doctors. The Bristol Stool Chart is widely recognized in medical practice. Stools categorized as levels 1 and 2 indicate constipation, levels 3–5 are considered within normal limits, and stools 6–7 are classified as very soft. Explain to patients that sometimes they may have stools that are a level 1–2 and that if they were constipated, softer stools may be behind these stools. Having softer stools after hard ones normally does not signify typical diarrhea; it indicates that they were constipated beforehand. This distinction can be hard for youth and parents to understand, but it is important as sometimes their doctors prescribe medication, patients take it, and start having loose stools. After starting medication, patients may pass loose stools and mistakenly believe the medication caused the diarrhea, when in fact it is helping resolve constipation by softening the stools. Most physicians suggest that if the stool remains soft for three or

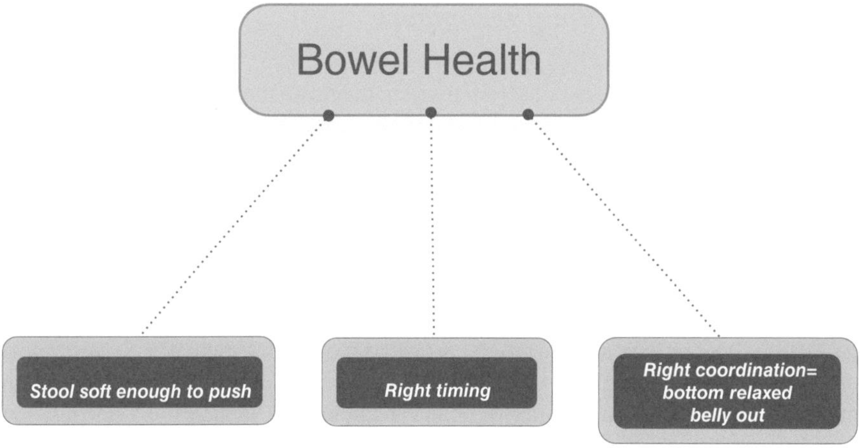

Fig. 22.2 Bowel health

more days, the medication dosage may be lowered or, in some cases, stopped. Close medical supervision is essential for proper medication management.

2. **Toilet Sitting at the Right Time:**

   For most patients, 'sitting at the right time' means responding to a natural bodily signal to use the toilet. However, when a patient is significantly constipated and their bowel has expanded, they may not receive this body signal to toilet sit. Gastrointestinal (GI) doctors often recommend that constipated individuals should aim to void at least once per day. If the patient is not receiving a signal to void daily or is not voiding daily, it is recommended that they toilet sit at set times. Often, toilet sitting about 20–60 min after meals can be helpful, while others may find it helpful to toilet sit after school or before bed. Based on patient interviews, if the patient is not getting a body signal, it is recommended that a treatment plan is made for the patient to toilet sit 3 times per day at times developed with the OT and patient. A chart can be developed to monitor toilet sitting, toilet sitting times, and stool type (Bristol level and size) {Fig 22.4, Appendix N]}.

3. **Right Coordination:**

   Even when a patient's stool is soft enough to pass and they are responding to body signals to void, improper coordination of pelvic and lower abdominal muscles can prevent complete bowel emptying. If a patient co-contracts these muscles while attempting to void, they may struggle to fully empty their bowels. A helpful tool for improving voiding posture is a foot stool that raises the knees to the level of, or above, the belly button. For younger children, a taller stool may be needed. An online resource, such as the educational version of the "Squatty Potty" video, explains the mechanics of why this foot stool is useful.

Appendix E: Toilet Sitting Techniques

Additionally, patients can benefit from training to ensure they are not co-contracting their lower abdominal muscles and the muscles adjacent to the anus. For patients with chronic constipation, they may benefit from outpatient pelvic floor biofeedback to address neuromuscular re-education. In such cases, electromyography (EMG) sensors are placed on the surface of the lower abdominal muscles and on the skin adjacent to the anus, allowing patients to see their muscle coordination on screen and learn to relax the pelvic muscles while activating the lower abdominal muscles.Though many inpatient and outpatient OTs may not have access to biofeedback equipment, education can still be provided to improve the patient's awareness of muscle coordination. Patients can be taught the importance of keeping the bottom muscles relaxed while activating their lower abdominal muscles. To do this, the occupational therapist can help the patient understand the correlation between the muscles in the legs and bottom. If the legs are relaxed by having soft knees (knees that can be moved if touched) and relaxed toes, then the bottom muscles are likely relaxed. One way to assess this is by ensuring the legs, knees, and toes are relaxed, which often correlates with relaxed pelvic muscles. At the same time, the lower abdominal muscles should be gently pushed outward. This technique is best practiced using diaphragmatic breathing, where the patient pushes the belly out while breathing in, and allows the stomach to stay out while still breathing.

This coordination exercise is ideally done in a simultaneous combination: bottom/legs/toes relaxed and belly out/activated for 20–30 s, then they should relax everything (including the stomach) for 30 s. Typically, this can be practiced for 5–10 reps (lower side for younger children) during their toilet sit times. There are some individuals who struggle to not co-contract their muscles. Having the "relax everything" for 30 s is important for these individuals, but it is important for everyone as individuals need breaks from coordinating their muscle groups (Fig. 22.3).

Toilet Sitting Techniques:

On the Toilet

★ Relax - Toes, Knees, Shoulders

Tummy Breathing
Breath in = tummy out
Breath out = tummy in

★ Breath in = tummy out and hold tummy out for 20 to 30 seconds (while breathing)
Relax for 20-30 seconds
Repeat up to 5-10 times

- Feet in "V" shape and knees out, relax bottom, knees, toes
- Test using hands to know where tummy muscles to use are
- Use footstool

Fig. 22.3 Toilet sitting techniques

Appendix F: Stool Log

When to Use a Stool Log

A stool log is typically recommended for individuals with chronic constipation issues, those who struggle to accurately report their stooling patterns to their doctor, or patients who have difficulty sharing this information with their parents. In many cases, parents are guided by GI doctors on how to adjust medications based on stool consistency and frequency, making accurate tracking crucial. For some patients, stooling feels quite private, and writing about it may be more comfortable than talking about it. Despite this, the patient may need some help to have a couple of stools examined by a health professional or parent to ensure they are correctly documenting them (see stool log figure) (Fig. 22.4, full size Appendix N).

Stool Log

	Sat	Sun	Mon	Tue	Wed	Thu	Fri	Sat	Sun	Mon	Tue	Wed	Thu	Fri	Sat	Sun	Mon	Tue	Wed	Thu	Fri
Enter date here-->																					
Morning																					
Sit in AM (yes or no)																					
BM? (S, M,L), BL																					
Afternoon																					
Sit in afternoon																					
BM? (S, M,L), BL																					
Sit after dinner																					
BM? (S, M,L), BL																					
Other Time BM																					
BM? (S, M,L), BL																					
Other Time BM																					
BM? (S,M,L), BL																					
Cup of hot water?																					

BM = Bowel Movement S = Small M = Medium L = Large

BL = Bristoll level (1-7) For other time BM, list time.

Fig. 22.4 Sample stool log

Appendix G: Chronic Pain Hand-Out

A visual that helps patients understand that those who are happiest with chronic pain tend to live life fully while not losing hope for a cure can help patients with chronic pain start to understand how to maximize their function while taking steps one at a time to see the impact on their pain (Fig. 22.5).

Sample Observation Log for Patient with Pain Issues

An observation log can be useful for patients with pain issues or issues related to sensations that are impacting their daily function. Notice that pain can be referred to as sensation to reframe if relevant. Categories can be modified and individualized per patient presentation (Fig. 22.6).

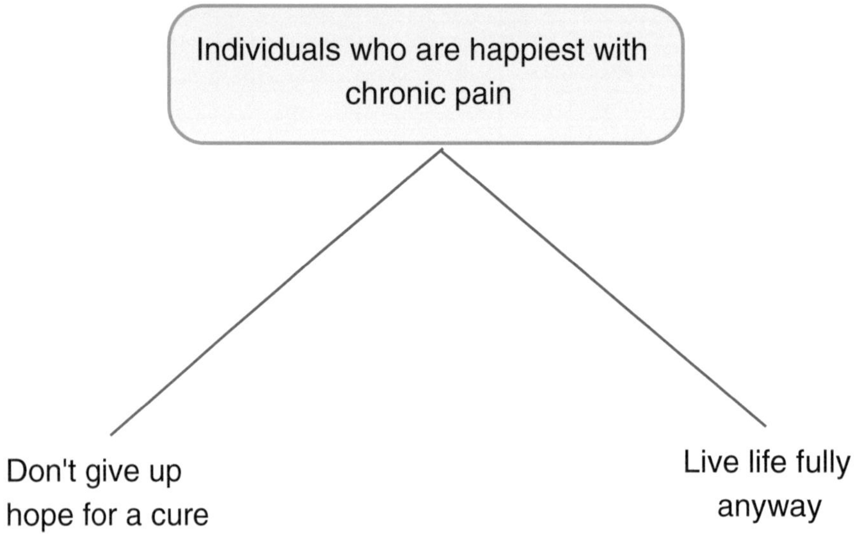

Fig. 22.5 Individuals with chronic pain

Observation Log: Please fill this log out every 30-60 waking minutes for 2-3 days or as directed by your team. After that you may fill it out when you notice something you want to share. Your team will assist you in examining any patterns.

Date/ Time	Nausea (1-10)	Stomach sensation (1-10)	Mood 1-10 1 word	Stress Level 1= least	Energy Level 1-10	Different factors (e.g., medication) outside time, activity, sleep	Hydration level 1-10 10= well hydrated	Current/ Upcoming activity	Productive Coping Strategy Used	Non-Productive Coping Tendency Used

Fig. 22.6 Observation log for patients with pain issues

Appendix H: Techniques for Addressing Throat Tightness

During feeding sessions, observe the patient's body and neck position carefully. **(Reference Video 7.12)**

Patients afraid of choking may raise their shoulders, tighten their neck, or unconsciously tuck their chin, which can hinder swallowing. Gentle redirection and education on maintaining a relaxed body posture and neutral chin position are beneficial.

Some patients with a fear of choking delay swallowing due to anxiety. Practicing the swallow process with fluids initially can help rebuild confidence.

While most patients do not delay swallowing liquids, those who do are encouraged to practice allowing liquid to naturally move to the back of the throat for immediate swallowing during therapy sessions. This practice can help rebuild confidence in the normal swallowing reflexes.

Teaching NUK brush exercises to these patients (see Chap. 7 and full-size available in Appendix N: Occupational Therapy-Developed Worksheets) can help them refresh their innate ability to chew and use their tongue. Remind them of the natural swallowing process: chewing food until ready to swallow, assisted by the tongue moving food to the back of the throat and into the esophagus [1]. Referencing this practice during the meal can help patients return to their prior eating ability.

Appendix I: Hydration

Goals can be set based on medical input for hydration. The below has a fill-in hydration chart that moves bottom to top. Each time the individual completes 4 oz, they color in their hydration block. This would be modified based on the individual patient's needs (Fig. 22.7).

Monday	Tuesday	Wednesday	Thursday	Friday	Saturday	Sunday
All met (5)	All met (5)	All met (5)	All met (5)	All met (5)	All met (5)	All met (5)
4 oz	4 oz	4 oz	4 oz	4 oz	4 oz	4 oz
4 oz	4 oz	4 oz	4 oz	4 oz	4 oz	4 oz
4 oz	4 oz	4 oz	4 oz	4 oz	4 oz	4 oz
4 oz	4 oz	4 oz	4 oz	4 oz	4 oz	4 oz
4 oz	4 oz	4 oz	4 oz	4 oz	4 oz	4 oz
4 oz	4 oz	4 oz	4 oz	4 oz	4 oz	4 oz
4 oz	4 oz	4 oz	4 oz	4 oz	4 oz	4 oz
4 oz	4 oz	4 oz	4 oz	4 oz	4 oz	4 oz
4 oz	4 oz	4 oz	4 oz	4 oz	4 oz	4 oz
4 oz	4 oz	4 oz	4 oz	4 oz	4 oz	4 oz

Fig. 22.7 Hydration chart sample

Appendix J: Sample Hydration Pacing Sheet and Instructions

Timed Fluid Sessions Sample

Below is a sample of a timed fluid session led initially by an occupational therapist, then RN supported and after a couple of days, parent supported

Sample Orders Related to Below Water trials

- RN to support pt in completing 12 oz of water at 10:15 a.m. over a 30 min period, 2 ounce per 5 min in AM and 2 oz per 5 min at 4 p.m. over a 30 min period. This is practice/treatment to support hydration/ prevent further need for IV
- Provide water in a full sized clear cup that indicates ounces so patient can see progress or mark it on his water bottle (either okay).
- Please utilize water target doc to support speed (see below behavior modification plan and copy kept in room)

Instructions for Using Chart

Please note that for the below document, a target completion time is set based on the start time. This document moves from top to bottom with the patient presented with the stated amount of fluid. Ahead of time, the occupational therapist sets goals for consumption quantity per time. The below sample included completing 2 oz over a 5 min period. Initially the patient started with a goal of 4 total ounces. Over time, it was increased to completing 12 ounces in one practice period. As skills were advanced, the level of support required decreased until the patient began spontaneously meeting his required fluid levels without support. Initially the patient had supported fluid times twice per day between meals (Fig. 22.8).

Fig. 22.8 Hydration pacing sheet

Water Target Document Start Time:

AM (2 oz/ 5 min)

	Listed on cup as:	Target Completion Time
12-10 oz		
10-8 oz		
8-6 oz		
6-4 oz		
4-2 oz		
2- 0 oz Done!		

Appendix K: Inpatient Feeding Plan Protocols and Processes for ARFID Patients

This appendix provides detailed protocols and workflow processes for managing inpatient feeding plans for ARFID patients, intended to help institutions implement or refine their own plans. The standard protocol for inpatients with anorexia nervosa-restricting subtype (AN-R) involves a strict meal schedule and nutrition replacement options. These patients typically follow a routine of three meals and two snacks each day, at our institution with breakfast at 8:30 a.m., lunch at 12:30 p.m., a snack at 2:30 p.m., dinner at 5:30 p.m., and a night snack at 8:30 p.m. Breakfast and snack periods are allocated 30 min, while lunch and dinner are allowed 40 min. After each meal and snack, patients are supervised for 1 h, during which time restroom access is restricted unless urgently needed. Any nutrition not consumed during meals or snacks is replaced with a liquid supplement or, if this is refused, is provided through a nasogastric (NG) tube.

In contrast, at our institution, ARFID patients often benefit from a modified approach that allows more flexibility and considers their specific needs. While structure and clarity remain important, the team typically avoids immediate use of the strict eat-replace protocol, especially for patients with a fear of aversive consequences. Instead, an ad lib plan is frequently more beneficial for these patients, allowing them to initially choose how much to eat and slowly work up to the required nutritional amount. The team has developed these ARFID-specific modifications through collaboration between occupational therapy (OT), nurse practitioners (NPs), registered dietitians (RDs), registered nurses (RNs), and other team members. This collaborative approach ensures the feeding plan is tailored to the patient's needs and adjusted based on progress. During team rounds and other discussions, the plan for the feeding orders may be refined or modified to better support the patient's recovery.

Occupational therapists are responsible for creating the initial feeding plan on the day of the OT evaluation and for updating the plan. The plan is bookmarked to allow easy access for all team members. Updates to the feeding plan are made as needed, with a new plan bookmarked replacing the previous one (by removing the bookmark) in the EHR each time it is updated. This ensures that the most current version is always available while maintaining a history of prior plans. If a paper chart is used, the plan can be updated manually, and a sticky tape bookmark can be placed to indicate the most up-to-date version. The related orders are entered into the electronic health record (EHR) by the NP. Nurses print and place the bookmarked plan on a clipboard, which is handed off between shifts to ensure continuity of care. When an update is made, the old plan is shredded, and the new one is used going forward.

Below is our feeding plan template, which demonstrates the sections that can be customized for each patient. While the format shown here is not editable, it illustrates the fields and structure used in the actual editable version maintained by the institution. This format ensures flexibility while maintaining consistent organization and clarity across all feeding plans.

Appendix L: Template for Bookmarked Feeding Plan

Reading This Template

- Selectable orders are in bold.
- Comments about how to choose the order are in regular text.
- Drop downs are indicated within angle brackets (i.e., < >).
- *** indicates a write in or an optional choice

OT Bookmarked Feeding Plan </Behavior Modification Plan>
Relevant Orders (Samples): ARFID

General

See OT Bookmarked Feeding Plan /<choice> Behavior Modification Plan

This is universally chosen; the Behavior Modification Plan section is only selected if there is an active behavior modification plan or Ladder Block Plan.

1:1 with core staff during all meals and snacks in room or on patio <drop down for other choice :>, 1:1 with core staff during all meals in room or on patio may attend group snacks.

This order is initially chosen for all patients to be 1:1 in their room or on the patio with staff. Once the patients have done training for three family meals with nursing and the family, this order is removed. Also, once the patient is doing well, snacks in groups may be tested. If that goes well this order may be completely removed as the patient may do meals in group when their family is not present. Many ARFID patients do better with eating when with 1:1 staff or with their families than eating in the group.

Pt can have *<45,60> min for all meals and* < 30,45,60> min for all snacks. If pt states they are done sooner <okay to end meal then, bring replacement at that time>.

The decision around this is based on the patient's baseline from the initial time you ate with them. For highly anxious patients, it is useful to provide more time so that the RN or milieu counselor eating with them does not rush them. This is especially important for fearful patients. Sometimes low-interest patients require more time at baseline to eat. Sometimes an additional piece of information is added here about when to bring replacement if it is relevant to the patient (e.g., 60 min for meal, bring replacement at 45 min).

Calorie count on daily cares flowsheet per meals and snacks and EPIC nursing note showing breakdown of calories consumed at each meal and snack for shift total. Provide behavioral observations regarding feeding tolerance and reported sensations

This is done for all patients that are ad lib or on a Ladder Block Plan, and often for patients on behavior modification plans.

Pt must attend all groups post meal

This is written when the structure of the group is anticipated to advance the patient's progress and the patient is not attending without extra encouragement.

Pt can keep food bedside

Often ARFID patients are allowed to trade in food items from home. Keeping some food bedside provides a convenient way to add items. For some patients (e.g., sensory eaters), it allows them to feel more secure knowing it is available. This is also relevant for patients who may need a carbonated drink.

Pt may use restroom at any time

This order is considered on a case-by-case basis. Some individuals with ARFID have fast digestion systems and tend to void post-eating. For individuals with issues of emesis, this order is not written, as the standard protocol is that patients cannot use the restroom for 1 hour after eating.

***(write in)**

It can be helpful for each section to have a write-in area **Mealtime Guidelines**

10:30 a.m. Snack daily

This is frequently added in the early phase for ARFID-fearful patients as they may not have much intake at once, providing more practice and opportunities for intake. It is also added for patients who may have issues with early satiety, which is common among ARFID-low interest patients. Sometimes for young patients with early bedtimes that are disrupted by night snack, an AM snack is added and a night snack is removed.

Lunch at < 11:45 a.m., 12 p.m.> daily (early tray). Please plan for vitals at 11 a.m.

Lunch may be started earlier when the patient doesn't have a morning snack, gets full easily, and can benefit from a larger gap between lunch and snack as they are scheduled close together. This is also added when the patient has up to 60 min for lunch.

Pt to sit up during all meals/snacks

This is common, but on admission, patients may eat in their bed on the first day when on bed rest, so this order is specified. If someone has a fear of vomiting or postural issues, this is an important order.

Pt to sit up during all meals/snacks ***<and 30 min post.;*** **Encourage feet on floor, relaxed posture, and abdominal breathing.> No vitals at that time.**

This order gets chosen if the patient has a strong fear of vomiting or vomiting issues.

***(write in)**

Feeding Plan/Supplementation/Replacement

No replacement required. Ad lib food. Document what is completed in nursing note. Calorie count.

This is a common order for fearful patients. It is often initially placed for sensory eaters as many do not tolerate the liquid supplement's taste. It is least common for ARFID-low interest patients as they typically can tolerate the supplement.

Pt may have unlimited optionals/trade foods and may receive credit for these items against required replacement. Okay to estimate.

This is a common initial order unless the patient does not demonstrate any preferred foods when filling out the Five guide preferred food list.

If supplementation is needed use: <specify supplement type *>.

This specifies the supplementation type.

Replacement is max * ml <has replacement type> even if pt has not completed full nutrition.**

A max replacement level is chosen if the patient has issues with vomiting or a fear of vomiting. Sometimes it is also chosen when a patient has sensory issues.

Initial replacement with *<supplement type>,* Initial replacement is a calorie replacement used with a supplement.

Mealtime Guidelines

10:30 a.m. Snack daily

This is frequently added in the early phase for ARFID-fearful patients as they may not have much intake at once, providing more practice and opportunities for intake. It is also added for patients who may have issues with early satiety, which is common among ARFID-low interest patients. Sometimes for young patients with early bedtimes that are disrupted by night snack, an AM snack is added and a night snack is removed.

Lunch at < 11:45 a.m., 12 p.m.> daily (early tray). Please plan for vitals at 11 a.m.

Lunch may be started earlier when the patient doesn't have a morning snack, gets full easily, and can benefit from a larger gap between lunch and snack as they are scheduled close together. This is also added when the patient has up to 60 min for lunch.

Pt to sit up during all meals/snacks

This is common, but on admission, patients may eat in their bed on the first day when on bed rest, so this order is specified. If someone has a fear of vomiting or postural issues, this is an important order.

Pt to sit up during all meals/snacks *<and 30 min post.;* Encourage feet on floor, relaxed posture, and abdominal breathing.> No vitals at that time.

This order gets chosen if the patient has a strong fear of vomiting or vomiting issues.

***(write in)

Feeding Plan/Supplementation/Replacement

No replacement required. Ad lib food. Document what is completed in nursing note. Calorie count.

This is a common order for fearful patients. It is often initially placed for sensory eaters as many do not tolerate the liquid supplement's taste. It is least common for ARFID-low interest patients as they typically can tolerate the supplement.

Pt may have unlimited optionals/trade foods and may receive credit for these items against required replacement. Okay to estimate.

This is a common initial order unless the patient does not demonstrate any preferred foods when filling out the Five guide preferred food list.

If supplementation is needed use: <E+, Lutrish (X.85 E+, *>.

This specifies the supplementation type.

Replacement is max * ml <has replacement type> even if pt has not completed full nutrition.**

A max replacement level is chosen if the patient has issues with vomiting or a fear of vomiting. Sometimes it is also chosen when a patient has sensory issues.

Initial replacement with *<supplement type>*, Initial replacement is a calorie replacement used with a supplement.

It's not uncommon for ARFID patients to use some alternate supplements from the AN population. This order specifies the supplement type.

****Pt to have *** mL <supplement type>, at each meal and snack. Bring at the start of the meal/snack and encourage pt to complete each time.**

The standard AN protocol is that replacement is brought at the end of the meal. If, while taste-testing the supplement, the patient struggles with drinking it, this order is often set to help the patient build the skill of taking the supplement at each meal and snack. Having the capacity to do so is also one of the prerequisites to the Ladder Block Plan and provides patients with additional nutritional options which can help with meeting nutritional goals.

*****(write in)**

Ladder Block Plan

Not Applicable at this time

This is the chosen drop down when the Ladder Block Plan is not being used.

Block value= * kcals, ***# of blocks today/ Block value increased on // at : p.m.**

This helps the nurses know the number of blocks and when the block value increases. Often, the block value (caloric value) is not increased until rounds, which means breakfast will have the prior block value whereas the snacks and meals post breakfast will have the increased value.

Pt has ladder block plan. Pt. may receive credit for blocks through provided food, optionals/ food from home, okay to estimate kcals. Please assist pt in trade-in options/liquid supplementation to make the blocks. Please do not replace above block value.

This order reviews the methods in which the patient can "make their block value," including presented food, food from home, and supplementation. Depending on the patient, they may receive nutrition that supersedes the caloric requirements to provide more options. It is important that the nurses do not supplement above the block value as this can result in patients feeling too full. However, sometimes patients spontaneously eat more, which is fine.

If patient completes extra kcals at any meal, it can be documented on Ladder Block Plan Extra kcal section and applied to future blocks.

As explained in the Ladder Block Plan section, overages are documented at the bottom and can be applied to future blocks if needed.

Pt is not on an eat-replace plan. Pt only needs the amount of nutrition of their blocks for each meal and snack even if there is more nutrition on the tray. Only provide the needed amount to make the block (or patient can choose other food items).

This is a bit redundant, but the RNs find it helpful. It reminds the RNs not to replace/supplement above the block value.

Calorie count on daily cares flowsheet per meals and snacks and EPIC nursing note showing breakdown of calories consumed at each meal and snack for shift total. Indicate blocks met. Provide behavioral observations regarding feeding tolerance and reported sensations.

The nurses record an EPIC note that specifies the calories consumed at each meal and snack. This information assists the OT in examining patterns and how to advance the patient's blocks or block value.

Please train patient and caregiver on use of the block plan. Please guide them through making calculations with their devices and using nutritional sheet to determine how pt is meeting her blocks.

Though the Ladder Block Plan becomes intuitive, it requires some initial training to learn how to use it effectively. The team works with the family to understand how to use the Ladder Block Plan.

Assist pt or family in completing ladder block document in room (drop down out of room) post each meal and snack.

Typically, the calculations for the Ladder Block Plan are done in the room. However, there are times where, due to the patient's young age or concern from the broader team about the negative impact of focusing on calories in front of the patient, all calculations are done outside the room and within the room values are only presented as "blocks" and not "calories."

Per bmod, if pt meets goals, pt may go to gift shop 1/day for 20 min w/ staff < in WC, while walking>.

As part of a reward plan, if parents choose that the patient earns money, they may visit the Stanford giftshop up to 1/day with staff. The walk is slightly longer, so at times wheelchair use is required.

(write in)

Behavior Modification (Not Ladder Block)

Not applicable at this time.

If a behavior modification (bmod) plan is not in use, this is marked as not applicable.

Follow behavior modification plan by OT. See OT bookmarked note.

This indicates that there is an individualized bmod plan.

Per bmod, if pt meets goals, pt may go to gift shop 1/day for 20 min w/ staff < in WC, while walking>.

As part of a reward plan, if parents choose that the patient earns money, they may visit the tanford giftshop up to 1/day with staff. The walk is slightly longer, so at times wheelchair use is required.

Assist pt or family in completing bmod document in room post each meal and snack.

This helps the family develop the skill and routine of completing the behavior modification document post meals.

*****(write in)**

Vomiting or Ruminating Patient

Separate food from fluids. No extra water on tray. Encourage water only prior to 30 min before meal or 1 h post meal.

Often, the nurses will move the patient's water bottle to the corner of the room or remove it during periods when the patient is not supposed to have fluid.

2 h a-code

A-code can be done (if approved) by the parent, within a group, or by any staff member. This supports the patient in breaking their vomiting or rumination patterns.

***(write in)

Challenge/Newer Foods

Not applicable.

Pt to use OT Food Exploration Log. See OT Bookmarked note for details.

This is for patients who use the food exploration log.

If patient has a newer food or a food they have not eaten before, please have them taste trial it at the start of the meal while filling out OT Food Exploration Log.

Within our institution, the RD indicates on the meal ticket (and on an additional spreadsheet if they are on the Ladder Block Plan) which foods are considered newer challenge foods. The OT, RN, or family member supports the patient in eating those foods first while using the food exploration log.

Pt does not need to replace RD documented challenge foods (listed on bottom of meal ticket).

At times the patient's plan calls for replacement, and at other times it does not. Challenge/newer foods are never replaced but if the patient has a Ladder Block Plan or is allowed trade foods, they may receive credit for what is consumed against replacement.

*(**write in**)

Family Meals

Please start family meals.

The nurses share an ARFID feeding hand-out and conduct a minimum of three meals with the patient and parents to support the FBT method of feeding their child.

1:1 with core staff during all meals and snacks in room until family is signed off.

Once family meals are completed, the patient may have meals with a trained family member. If a trained family member is not present, provide 1:1 with core staff in the room or on the patio.

***(**write in**)

The below section does not consist of orders, it has the patient identification and feeding tips. For ease of reading, the template is placed in bold and comments are not bold.

Identification:

Pt is a * y/o {female/male/non-binary} with diagnosis of <ARFID - Fear of aversive consequences, ARFID - Avoidance based on sensory characteristics of food, ARFID - Low interest, ED NOS>, and ***. Pt presents with <nausea, fear of nausea, emesis, fear of vomiting, rumination, stomach pain, feeling "too full", fear of choking, limited food variety, oral-motor weakness, immature oral motor patterns, sensory sensitivity to food> significantly impacting ability to achieve adequate nutritional intake. Pt identifies barriers to eating as ***. *****

For the above, the occupational therapist gets information from the psychology team about the patient's subtype and identifying factors. The occupational therapist evaluation provides information about the patient's barrier and perceived barriers.

Feeding Tips

- **Keep topics neutral (off school, off family). Pt has a variety of interests: *****

The above is consistently chosen as a feeding tip.

Drop Down Choices for Additional Feeding Tips

**<- Encourage pt to sit in chair during mealtime

- **Please complete challenge foods (as listed on RD meal ticket) first while pt still has an appetite. Please assist pt in logging these on OT Food Exploration Log.**
- **If pt is reporting nausea/looks nauseated, encourage relaxed posture (feet on ground, relaxed knees, relaxed shoulders) and abdominal breathing.**
- **If pt is reporting nausea/looks nauseated, may suggest using nausea relief band.**
- **Pt may watch media/listen to music during the meal.***>**

Appendix M: Bookmarked Feeding Plan Sample with Progression

OT Bookmarked Feeding Plan Sample

Below is one sample progression of the order section of the bookmarked OT Feeding Plan.

SAMPLE FEEDING PLAN PROGRESSION FOR A SHORT STAY (3 total days), FEAR OF AVERSIVE CONSEQUENCE PATIENT

Day 1 hospitalization fear of vomiting/ contamination with anticipated short stay. Of note this patient responded very well to the structure of the hospital with nursing support, immediately started eating all foods she had eliminated, tolerated supplementation well and was able to be advanced quickly.

OT Feeding Plan (Day 1)

** Please note patient plan likely to change each weekday. Please check daily. Updated orders are in **bold.**

General

- See OT Bookmarked Feeding Plan
- Please document calorie count/ patient behavioral patterns during meals in a nursing EPIC note.
- 1:1 with core staff until family is signed off for family meals

Mealtime Guidelines

- Lunch at 12pm daily (early tray). Please plan for vitals at 11am.
- Pt can sit in the chair for all meals and snacks and for 30 min post.

Feeding Plan/Supplementation/Replacement

- Pt to have 60ml 1.5+ kcal/mL supplement at each meal and snack. Bring at the start of meal/snack and encourage pt to complete each time.

Ladder Block Plan

- Not Applicable at this time.

Behavior Modification Plan (Not Ladder Block)

- Not Applicable at this time.

Vomiting or Ruminating Patient

- Not Applicable.

Challenge Foods

- Not Applicable.

Family Meals

- Please start family meals.

Identification Patient is an 10-year old female with a hx of anxiety and constipation who presents with weight loss in the setting of restrictive eating due to fear of illness/vomiting with diagnosis of ARFID - Fear of aversive consequences. Pt presents with fear of vomiting and fear of food poisoning significantly impacting ability to achieve adequate nutritional intake. Pt identifies barriers to eating as feeling fearful she will vomit, concern over what to eat (i.e., notes that aunt is a "vegetarian" and pt. concern about food positioning). Pt has several checking behaviors and often requires food to be bought the same day in order to eat it.

Feeding Tips
- Keep topics neutral (off school, off family). Pt has a variety of interests: her kitten, painting
- Encourage pt to sit in chair during mealtime
- If pt is reporting nausea/looks nauseated, encourage relaxed posture (feet on ground, relaxed knees, relaxed shoulders) and abdominal breathing.
- If patient is hesitant about starting a food, please encourage her "to practice taking bites."

Behavior Modification Plan/Log System Instructions
- Not Applicable at this time.

Behavior Modification Plan/Log
- Not Applicable at this time.

Day 2 and Homegoing Plan

Of note, patient had tolerated 2 ounces of a 1.5 supplement for 24 h, was taking over 1000 kcals and her parents were interested in a Ladder Block Plan that they could use to track her caloric intake. The patient was young so the parents did not want to "talk calories" in the room, therefore all discussions about calories took place outside of her hospital room and within the room they just let her know "if she made her blocks." Whenever the plan is updated, changes are made in bold. Cross outs can also be used.

OT Feeding Plan and Ladder Block Plan

** Please note patient plan likely to change each weekday. Please check daily. Updated orders are in **bold.**

General
- See OT Bookmarked Feeding Plan
- Please document calorie count/ patient behavioral patterns during meals in a nursing EPIC note.

- **Pt can have 45 min for all meals and 30 min for all snacks. If pt states they are done sooner support in meeting blocks or end meal if blocks are met.**

Mealtime Guidelines

- Lunch at 12pm daily (early tray). Please plan for vitals at 11am.
- Pt can sit in the chair for all meals and snacks and for 30 min post.

Feeding Plan/Supplementation/Replacement

- NA, if pt requests some supplementation, please use boost strawberry

Ladder Block Plan

- **Block value= 300 kcals per block. 7# of blocks today., pt plan today starts from lunch.**
- **Pt has ladder block plan. Pt may receive credit for blocks through provided food, optionals/food from home, okay to estimate kcals. Please assist pt in trade-in options/liquid supplementation to make the blocks. Please do not replace above block value.**
- **Pt is not on an eat-replace plan. Pt only needs the amount of nutrition of their blocks for each meal and snack even if there is more nutrition on the tray. Only provide the needed amount to make the blocks (or patient can choose other food items).**
- **Calorie count on daily cares flowsheet per meals and snacks and EPIC nursing note showing breakdown of calories consumed at each meal and snack for shift total. Indicate blocks met. Provide behavioral observations regarding feeding tolerance and reported sensations.**
- **Please train pt and caregiver on use of the ladder block plan. Please guide them through making calculations with their devices and using nutritional sheet to determine how pt is meeting their blocks.**
- **Assist pt or family in completing ladder block plan in room post each meal and snack.**
- **Pt is young. Please do not talk about calories or caloric block value in front of patient. If she gets extra calories over the blocks, please support family in documenting it as block fractions (e.g., 1/10, 1/2 block, etc.) rather than in calorie value.**

Behavior Modification Plan (Not Ladder Block)

- Not Applicable at this time.

Vomiting or Ruminating Patient

- Not Applicable.

Challenge Foods

- **Pt has a place on her ladder block plan where she is documenting "newer foods." These include foods that she has not eaten in a month or more or a completely new food that she tries.**

Family Meals

- Please start family meals.

Identification Patient is an 10-year old female with a hx of anxiety and constipation who presents with weight loss in the setting of restrictive eating due to fear of illness/vomiting with diagnosis of ARFID—Fear of aversive consequences. Pt presents with fear of vomiting and fear of food poisoning significantly impacting ability to achieve adequate nutritional intake. Pt identifies barriers to eating as feeling fearful she will vomit, concern over what to eat (I.e., notes that aunt is a "vegetarian" and concern about food positioning). Pt has several checking behaviors and often requires food to be bought the same day in order to eat it.

Feeding Tips

- Keep topics neutral (off school, off family). Pt has a variety of interests: her kitten, painting
- Encourage pt to sit in chair during mealtime
- If pt is reporting nausea/looks nauseated, encourage relaxed posture (feet on ground, relaxed knees, relaxed shoulders) and abdominal breathing.
- If patient is hesitant about starting a food, please encourage her "to practice taking bites."

Behavior Modification Plan/ Log System Instructions

- Each meal/ snack block represents "a block of nutrition" per RD guidelines of specific caloric value/ block.
- Please color block Green when completed at meal, Yellow when completed at a later meal.
- Please note that coloring the full amount in green represents getting all required nutrition at that mealtime with any nutritional source.
- Food items may be exchanged or replaced with other food items or supplement (if desired).
- It is important to keep rotating food items to avoid food jags.
- If more block value is achieved during a meal than the block needs, record the extra value in the bottom "extra blocks" section, they may be used to complete later blocks as needed/desired (within the same day only).
- Only color in complete block(s) if that full nutritional value is consumed at that meal or used in combination with the "extra kcal" calories. When those are used, cross them off to indicate they have been utilized.
- If blocks are not fully completed at any meal, color only up to what has been completed, leaving that section blank, if made up later (by going over at a subsequent meal or snack and giving caloric credit), color in yellow.
- Always first color the blocks for that meal/ snack before making up nutrition from a prior meal.

Appendix N: Occupational Therapy-Developed Worksheets

Productive Coping Strategies
Physiological Recovery Model
Bowel Health
Toilet Sitting Techniques
Stool Log
Individuals with chronic pain
NUK Brush Exercises
Step-by-Step Food Exploration Log
Step-by-Step Food Exploration Log & Reward Chart

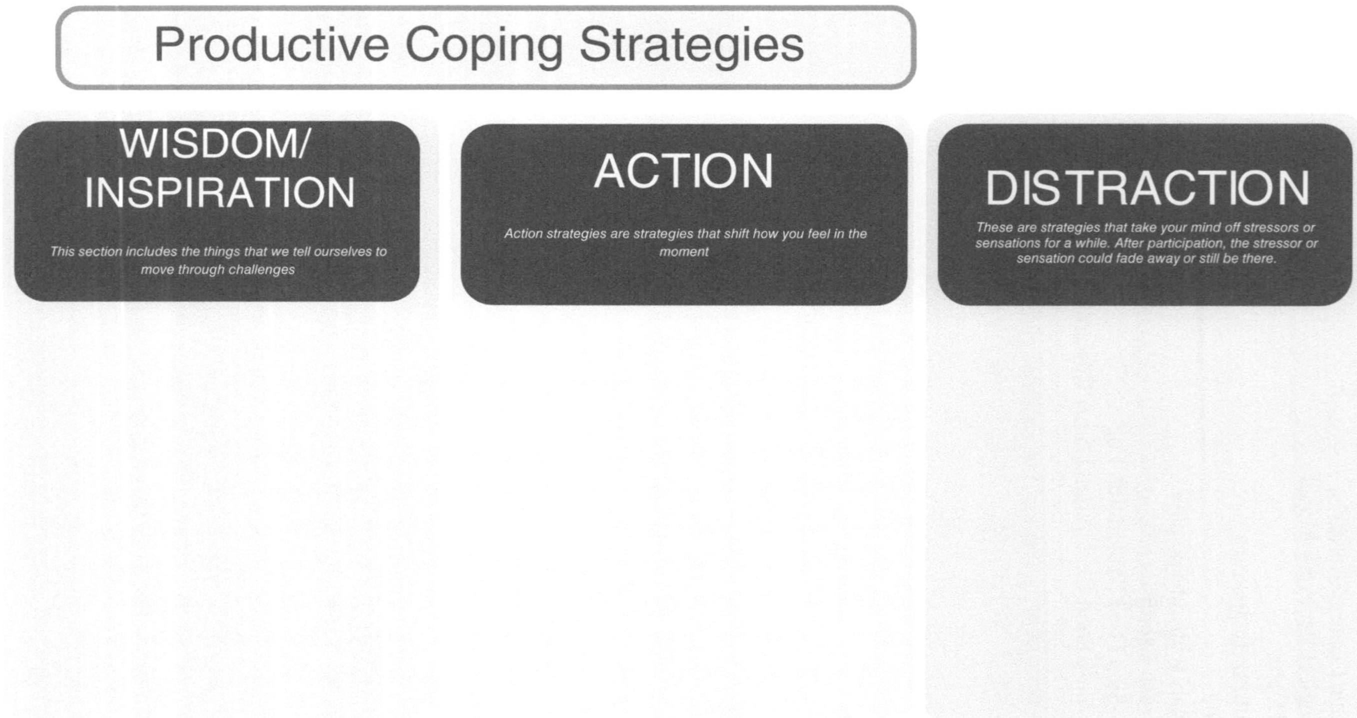
Productive Coping Strategies
WISDOM/ INSPIRATION
This section includes the things that we tell ourselves to move through challenges
ACTION
Action strategies are strategies that shift how you feel in the moment
DISTRACTION
These are strategies that take your mind off stressors or sensations for a while. After participation, the stressor or sensation could fade away or still be there.

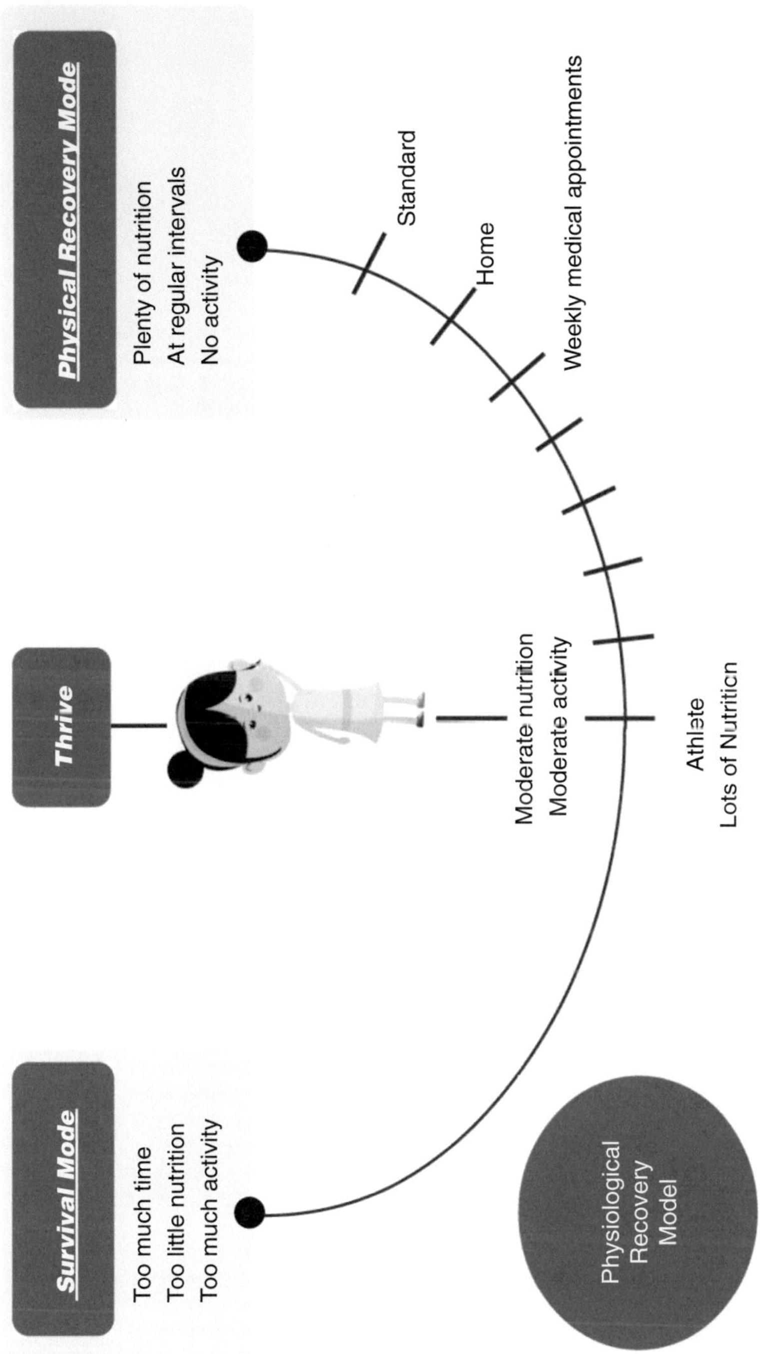
Physical Recovery Mode
Plenty of nutrition
At regular intervals
No activity
Standard
Home
Weekly medical appointments
Thrive
Moderate nutrition
Moderate activity
Athlete
Lots of Nutrition
Survival Mode
Too much time
Too little nutrition
Too much activity
Physiological Recovery Model

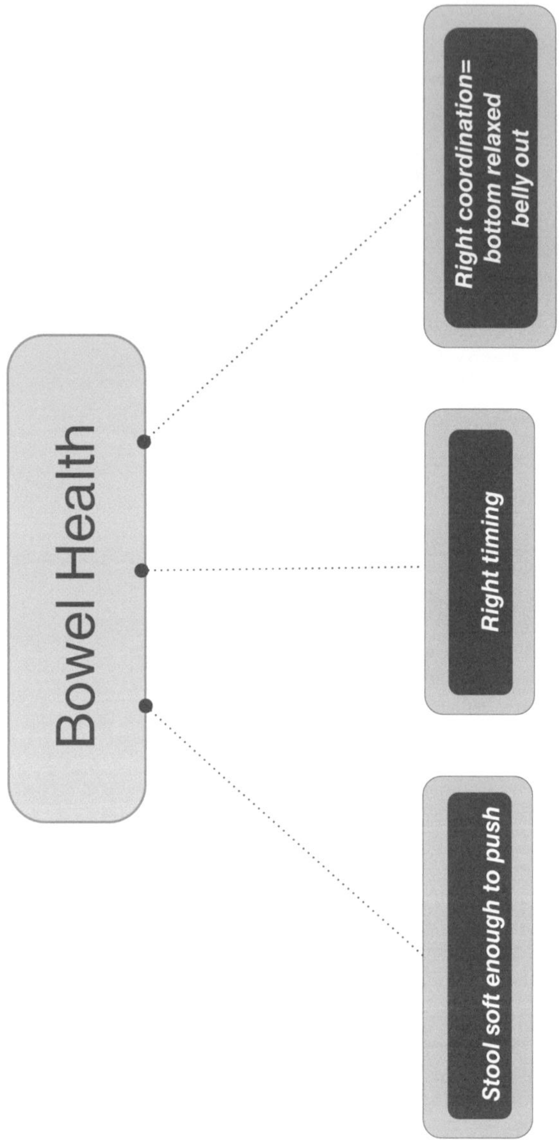
Bowel Health
Right coordination= bottom relaxed belly out
Right timing
Stool soft enough to push

Toilet Sitting Techniques:

On the Toilet

★ Relax - Toes, Knees, Shoulders

Tummy Breathing
Breath in = tummy out
Breath out = tummy in

★ Breath in = tummy out and hold tummy out for 20 to 30 seconds (while breathing)
Relax for 20-30 seconds
Repeat up to 5-10 times

- Feet in “V” shape and knees out, relax bottom, knees, toes
- Test using hands to know where tummy muscles to use are
- Use footstool

Stool Log

	Sat	Sun	Mon	Tue	Wed	Thu	Fri	Sat	Sun	Mon	Tue	Wed	Thu	Fri	Sat	Sun	Mon	Tue	Wed	Thu	Fri
Enter date here-->																					
Morning																					
Sit in AM (yes or no)																					
BM? (S, M,L), BL																					
Afternoon																					
Sit in afternoon																					
BM? (S, M,L), BL																					
Sit after dinner																					
BM? (S, M,L), BL																					
Other Time BM																					
BM? (S, M,L), BL																					
Other Time BM																					
BM? (S,M,L), BL																					
Cup of hot water?																					

BM = Bowel Movement S = Small M = Medium L = Large

BL = Bristoll level (1-7) For other time BM, list time.

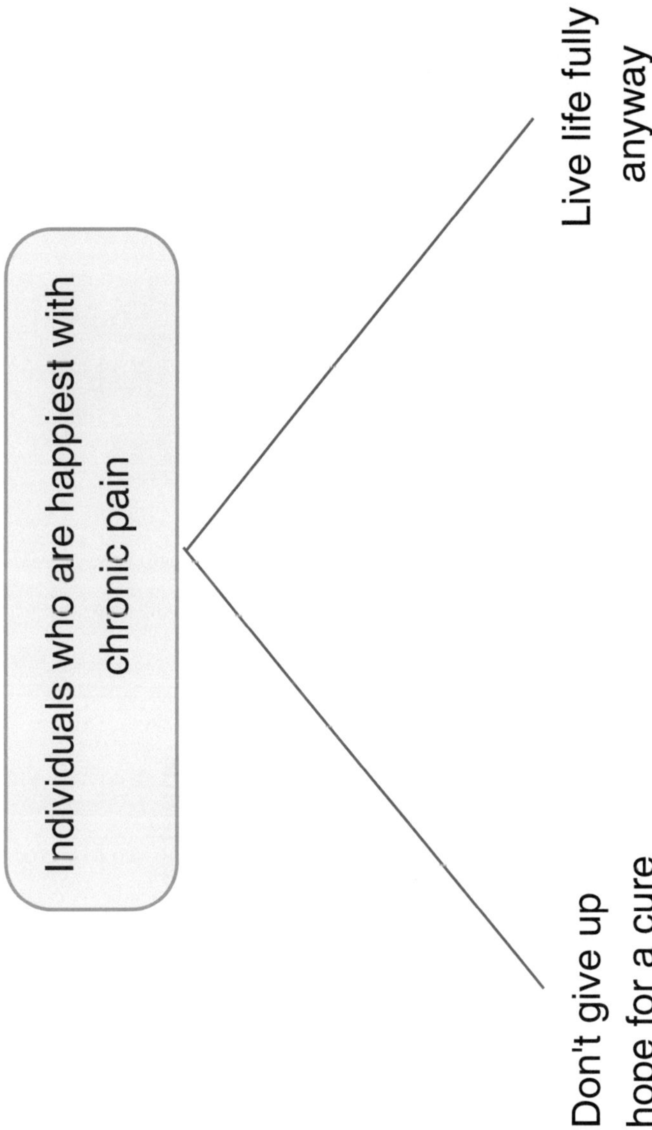
Individuals who are happiest with chronic pain
Don't give up hope for a cure
Live life fully anyway

Oral Motor Exercises

- **With nuk brush, place inside of mouth, chew strong x10**
- **Move brush to other side only with tongue**

Repeat 10 reps, 5 on each sides of the mouth

- **Last 2 times, pull softly + hold using resistance to keep nuk brush in place**

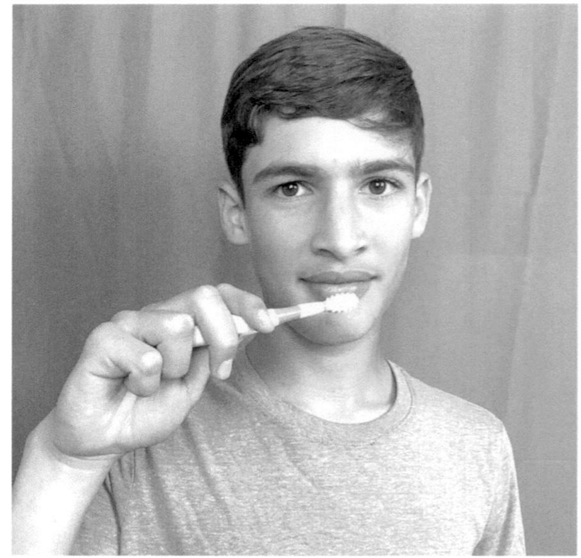

Directions for Food Exploration Log: (Record all answers on log, when possible, staff or family should fill out the log so that the patient can focus on eating).
- Prior to starting, patient's food to be explored and preferred change-taste food/drink and a drink should be in front of them. Review what change-taste taste food item is (i.e., an enjoyed item to change the flavor of the food).
- Newer foods should be trialed at the start of the meal, prior to any other item.
- Have individual with ARFID first rank appearance prior to taking a bite. 0= looks terrible, 5= looks great, 3= in the middle.
- Review that the first bite will be to rank texture, 0-5, 0= terrible texture, 5= great texture, 3= in the middle.
- Let them know the next bite is a ranking of flavor. 0= terrible flavor, 5= great flavor, 3 = in the middle.
- Let them know the next bite is for ranking "like it." 0= do not like it at all, 5= like it a lot, 3= in the middle.
- Ask, do you think you would try it again on another day? Yes, No, Maaaybe? It's good to extend the maybe out as it often helps them consider it more. If they disliked it, consider saying, "Do you think you would try it in a different form (e.g., crunchier, more cooked, with a dip, etc.)?"
-If the food has been trialed before, indicate how many times in "Trial of this Food #"

Step-by-Step Food Exploration Log

(to support growth, health, energy and a full life)

Please have at least 3 bites of a newer food at meals and/or snacks and rank 1- 5 below. Take a bite to explore texture, a bite to explore flavor and a bite to explore "like it."

Date	Item Name	Appearance 0-5	Texture 0-5	Flavor 0-5	Like it 0-5	Do you think you try it again on a different day? (Yes, no, maybe)	Quantity eaten:	Trial of this Food #

Directions for Food Exploration Log: (Record all answers on log, when possible, staff or family should fill out the log so that the patient can focus on eating).
- Prior to starting, patient's food to be explored and preferred change-taste food/drink and a drink should be in front of them. Review what change-taste taste food item is (i.e., an enjoyed item to change the flavor of the food).
- Newer foods should be trialed at the start of the meal, prior to any other item.
- Have individual with ARFID first rank appearance prior to taking a bite. 0= looks terrible, 5= looks great, 3= in the middle.
- Review that the first bite will be to rank texture, 0-5, 0= terrible texture, 5= great texture, 3= in the middle.
- Let them know the next bite is a ranking of flavor. 0= terrible flavor, 5= great flavor, 3 = in the middle.
- Let them know the next bite is for ranking "like it." 0= do not like it at all, 5= like it a lot, 3= in the middle.
- Ask, do you think you would try it again on another day? Yes, No, Maaaybe? It's good to extend the maybe out as it often helps them consider it more. If they disliked it, consider saying, "Do you think you would try it in a different form (e.g., crunchier, more cooked, with a dip, etc.)?"
-Indicate point value earned in last column. Clarify what points are used for at bottom of document (individualize per patient)

Step-by-Step Food Exploration Log & Reward Chart

(to support growth, health, energy and a full life)

Please have at least 3 bites of a challenge food at meals and/or snacks and rank 1- 5 below. Take a bite to explore texture, a bite to explore flavor and a bite to explore "like it."

Date	Item Name	Appearance 0-5	Texture 0-5	Flavor 0-5	Like it 0-5	Do you think you try it again on a different day? (Yes, no, maybe)	Quantity eaten:	Took 3 bites or more= 1 point, List points

SAMPLE POINT IDEAS, CHOICE ONE (OR DIFFERENT) AND UTILIZE

1 point = (sample ideas) 10 min game time – or- 5 pts = $1 per chosen activity -or- 3 pt = choice activity (e.g., choosing movie, outing, dinner, etc.)

Reference

1. Thomas S, Sauter W, Starrost U, Pohl M, Mehrholz J. Regaining water swallowing function in the rehabilitation of critically ill patients with intensive-care-unit acquired muscle weakness. Disabil Rehabil. 2018;40(13):1494–500. https://doi.org/10.1080/09638288.2017.1300341.

Index

A. B. Sinha et al., *Comprehensive Clinical Care for Adolescents with Avoidant/Restrictive Food Intake Disorder (ARFID)*,
https://doi.org/10.1007/978-3-031-92232-9